"A thorough and well written discussion of the questions which arise before, during and after menopause. It is written in clear and adult language, without patronizing the reader."

—Anonymous

"This book will give courage to the suggestion of taking charge of our own health and not treating it as a sickness but a moving on to better and different things. A lot of myths were dispelled and new information given that will make the transition a more comfortable and positive moving forward."

—Donna Lenhardt
Danville, California

"The text moved smoothly from past to present to future and guides one through and informs one of what has happened, what is happening and what will happen. It is aimed at the young, the old, the female, and the male."

—Mary Ellen Haithcock
Alamo, California

"Research chapter was informative and welcome and covered many facets of information not readily available to the public."

—Paula Thompson
Concord, California

"This is a book that fills in many blanks of information about the difference between the care of men and women as to diet, exercise, heart conditions, and chemical imbalance."

—Anonymous

"This book is informative, comprehensive, inclusive, factual and instructional regarding bodily changes a woman might expect as she goes through the phases of premenopause, menopause and postmenopause."

—Genevieve Layng
Casselberry, Florida

"I wish I would have been introduced to a book such as this when I was young so I could have prepared ahead for menopause. This was never talked about. Thanks for informing the women of yesterday, today and tomorrow. Even though I have some medical knowledge I didn't realize the importance of preparing for menopause."

—Marge Schantner
Elm Grove, Wisconsin

"I wish I'd had this book 15 years ago. How much easier it would have been going through the menopause years. As is, I fumbled my way through the stages—confused—uninformed—misinformed. Had I had this book I would have saved myself many embarrassing moments. I was one of those women with hot flashes/flushes that never quit. I hate to think of all the water that ran off my face and down my back at the most inopportune times."

—Helen Frank
Lincoln City, Oregon

"I really enjoyed reading this book. I've learned a lot and I'm more informed about menopause and other health issues that face us now and as we age."

—Patti Buschke
Milwaukee, Wiscon

"This is an exceptionally informative and comprehensive guide for intelligent and educated women, providing answers to many common questions about menopause and aging."

—Mona M. Shangold, M.D., F.A.C.O.G., F.A.C.S.M.
Co-Author of The Complete Sports
Medicine Book for Women

"An invaluable resource for women who want current, understandable information about how to transition through the years before and after menopause in the healthiest way possible."

—Susan B. Moskosky, M.S., R.N.C.
Bethesda, Maryland

Today and Tomorrow's Woman

Today and Tomorrow's Woman

Menopause: Before and After
(Girls of 16 to Women of 99)

Virginia Layng Millonig, Ph.D. R.N.

Health Leadership Associate's Inc.
Potomac, Maryland

HEALTH LEADERSHIP ASSOCIATES, INC.
Manuscript Editor   Susan Moskosky
Medical Technical Writer   Mary Virginia Gray
Cover Design   Suzuki Graphic Design
Interior Design   Suzuki Graphic Design
Photography   Al Dintino
Production   Port City Press

Printed in the United States of America

Health Leadership Associates, Inc.
P.O. Box 59153
Potomac, Maryland 20859

Library of Congress Cataloging-in-Publication Data
Millonig, Virginia Layng.
    Today and tomorrow's woman: menopause—before and after:
girls of 16 to women of 99 / Virginia Layng Millonig.
        p. cm.
    Includes bibliographical references and index.
    ISBN 1-878028-23-5
    1. Menopause—Popular works. 2. Menopause—Complications—Prevention.
    3. Women—Health and hygiene. 4. Self-care, Health.
I. Title.
    RG186.M55   1996
    618.1'75—dc20   95-48849
                                                                              CIP

NOTICE: The author and publisher of this book have taken care that the information and recommendations contained herein are accurate and compatible with standards generally accepted at the time of publication. However, the author and publisher cannot and do not accept responsibility for errors or omissions, if any in this book, or for the consequences from application of the information in this text and they make no warranties, EXPRESS OR IMPLIED, with respect to the contents of the book.

How to Order: Copies may be ordered from Health Leadership Associates, Inc., P.O. Box 59153, Potomac, MD 20854; 1-800-435-4775. Quantity discounts are also available.

Contents

blood pressure; learn about prevention techniques to lower cholesterol and blood pressure, to stop smoking, to lose weight, and more.

Discuss hormone replacement therapy and its use during menopause; learn that using hormone replacement therapy is a personal decision; review types of hormones available and treatment schedules; consider the need for and problems associated with estrogen therapy; and review the effects of hormone replacement therapy on uterine and breast health; discuss alternatives to hormone replacement therapy.

Gain ideas on assuring good nutrition; maintaining a healthy weight; decreasing fat and cholesterol in the diet; moderating sugar, salt, and alcohol intake; developing a realistic and safe exercise program; and coping with stress.

Develop an awareness of the importance of research to the understanding of menopause and women's health; review past and current studies; appreciate the need for future studies.

Preface

All females must prepare for their future health much as they prepare for their future career goals in life, and probably of greatest importance is that this preparation for a continuous state of good health never stops.

Although there are several books available which focus on the menopausal period and beyond of a women's life, few take into account the time prior to menopause, even as early as the teen years. What is different about this book is that early steps to prevent problems, later on in life, are discussed in great detail. The audience for this book are women in their mid to late thirties, women in the menopause transition phase, and those for whom menopause is but a memory. It is even for the moms of those teenagers whose current lifestyles so dramatically affect their current and future health. Yes, even teenagers can develop osteoporosis! There is something for everyone including the men! Scientific information has been transformed into readable and understandable language to enable the reader to understand what is affecting her body at various stages in her lifetime. Ultimately, together with her health care professional, she will be able to make an informed decision regarding her own health care.

Many of the myths associated with the menopausal experience are explained including how various cultures view menopause. What menopause is not is further documented. A detailed description of various hormones and their effect on the female body is given starting with puberty. Many of the problems associated with the menopause and post-menopausal years such as hot flashes, urinary and sexual problems are covered as well as the treatment and solutions, but the most serious—osteoporosis and heart disease—are described in great detail as well as the steps to avoid them. Many of the controversies and alternatives for hormone replacment therapy are described. You will even find the latest on the breast cancer controversy.

There are major sections on how to avoid the pitfalls we all encounter as we age, and that is the weight accumulation. How to take care of weight problems including meal plans, how to shop and prepare foods to increasing one's metabolism is covered in the latter part of the book. Topics range from how to calculate fat intake to determining your target heart rate. You will even be able to tell how many calories you burn when you engage in different types of activities. A sample walking and jogging program is provided and the latest on exercise machines, both use and how to purchase them is included. An easy way to cope with the stress in your life is also covered. You will be amazed at the usefulness of this book which will make you an informed partner regarding your own health care.

And finally there is an entire chapter for those of you who want to know what kind of research has been conducted thus far in the area of women's health and what the results of the current studies will tell which will hopefully give us even better information.

The final addition to the book is an extensive resource list which can put you into contact with most every government agency and professional association that pertains to you as a woman with the latest accurate and scientific information you may want on any subject pertaining to the health of today and tomorrow's women.

Acknowledgements

This book reflects the input of a variety of individuals, agencies and associations. Their unique contributions are reflected throughout the book. I would like to especially thank Catherine Garner, DrPH., R.N.C., Patricia D. Kellogg, M.D., Susan B. Moskosky, MS., R.N.C., Veronica A. Ravnikar, M.D. and Mona M. Shangold, M.D., who generously gave their time and expertise. And a special thanks also to the many women who took the time and effort to help make this book one which will indeed make every woman who reads it an informed member of her own health care team.

Appreciation is extended to The National Osteoporosis Foundation, American Heart Association, Department of Health and Human Services, Department of Agriculture, National Institutes of Health, The Food and Drug Administration, National Heart, Lung and Blood Institute, and National Cancer Institute for their cooperation and assistance.

Introduction

TAKE CONTROL

Women have the hapless distinction of experiencing what is called the "Change of Life" or menopause. Although not a life change, menopause is a health event and requires adequate preparation in order to maintain a healthy body.

Knowledge provides the building blocks for sound planning. Information on menopause often filters through the mother-to-daughter link. The information passed through this chain must be purged of the myths and taboos associated with menopause and updated with knowledge based on medical research.

Women now can acquire accurate information that can aid them in communicating with their health care providers, their families, and most importantly other women. As with other women's health issues, only education and current medical knowledge will change the way both women and men view menopause.

Menopause is a celebration of experience earned and of the possibilities yet to come. A woman must prepare to meet her future with a strong and healthy body.

WOMEN TODAY

Women spend most of their lives managing what happens to others—their spouses, children, elderly parents—yet they have been unable to exercise the same control when it comes to issues that affect them directly, most specifically their health. Oddly enough in the area of health, women have either been treated just like men or their problems have been ignored. Fortunately today subjects like pregnancy, menstruation, fertility, and breast cancer are no longer topics worthy only of a back room discussion. Yet even with this new openness, women are still considered to be slaves to their bodies. Consider that a man's life is measured in productive years: childhood, education, employment, and retirement while a woman's life is measured in body cycles: childhood, puberty, childbearing years, menopause, and postmenopause. Each phase conjures up images of a woman controlled by hormonal rushes and body changes. Slowly, very slowly, the old notions that "female problems"must simply be endured are dissolving. Women's health issues are openly discussed and carry no shame. Yet the control women are asserting in other areas of their lives has not yet taken hold in the area of menopause.

Menopause is not a mysterious phenomenon that ruins the body and leaves it wasted. As with health in general, menopause can be managed and controlled with proper planning and healthy activities. Women can help themselves and each other by relying on facts and not the fiction pertaining to the menopausal process.

SOON YOU WILL BE IN CONTROL

Based upon the known facts and dilemmas surrounding menopause, this book has been written to assist and inform women about the entire menopausal experience. Common symptoms, trends and benefits of treatment, prevention of diseases such as osteoporosis and cardiovascular disease, as well as ways to keep women feeling great and wonderful will all be covered to provide answers and solutions to pertinent questions. In addition to critical information, the case is made for a prevention campaign that can and should begin early in life and continue through adolescence and young adulthood into the menopause period and beyond. Prevention techniques are discussed to allow women to become proactive participants in this event. Look also for a discussion of the latest research, and its applicability to women's health issues.

While written for women approaching menopause, experiencing the transition, or enjoying the postmenopausal state, health professionals involved in education and training should consider this book as a resource for their clients. All women have the right to be well informed about their bodies and the options available to help them maintain health and vigor. Women have much living to do!

DID YOU KNOW?

- Nearly one third of a woman's life is spent in the estrogen-deficient, postmenopausal state.

- A woman at age 50 with no unusual risk factors has a life expectancy of 82.8 years.

- In the 1900s, the average age of menopause was 51. Today that average age is still the same which means there is still a "lot of living" for women who approach the age of 50 years.

- Major problems of the postmenopausal period can be prevented by preparation during adolescence and the young adult years.

- Taking care of a hot flash is a very small part of the management of menopause.

- Although not for everyone, hormone replacement therapy has many advantages for both menopausal and postmenopausal women. Some advantages include the management of hot flashes, the prevention of fractures, and the maintenance of a healthy heart.

- Menopause does not end a woman's sexual life.

DO YOU KNOW?

- the normal signals of menopause,
- the not so normal signals of menopause; and
- that a woman need not be destined to a life of fractures, hot flashes, depression, and heart problems resulting from menopause.

ARE YOU?

- under 35 and feel menopause is somewhere on the horizon, but not an immediate concern,
- approaching menopause or in the transition phase when cycle irregularities and unpredictable episodes of heavy uterine bleeding occur; or
- one of those women who went through menopause recently, and feel it's over and done with and none of this menopause information is for you.

THIS BOOK IS FOR YOU

If you answered "yes" to any of the last three questions or do not have the answers to all the others, don't feel guilty. You are not alone. In spite of the fact that many women of today are well informed about their bodies, many are left with a variety of unanswered questions because of conflicting, confusing information.

After many years of conducting seminars for women, nurses, and other health professionals who managed the health of women, it became apparent that for most women the above questions and a myriad of others were a very real problem, and neither educational level, nor role seemed to make a difference.

Many of these women were uncertain of what was happening to their bodies, and many were reluctant, embarrassed, or for other reasons unable to get their questions answered. They were "starved" for knowledge regarding the reaction of their bodies to this life experience.

A BIT OF HISTORY

Fact Or Fiction

Separating menopause fact from fiction has never been an easy task because the information just did not exist. The idea that women's health issues may be different from men's health issues is fairly new, and the menopausal process is but a part of the larger field of women's health.

History And Health

The prior lack of concern for women's health issues corresponds to history's view of women as second class citizens. Higher education and medical schools bore this out as men outnumbered women in colleges and male medical students far outnumbered their female counterparts. Although the tide has turned with the enrollment of women surpassing men in many universities and colleges and female medical school enrollment increasing, the difference between men and women and their responses to various diseases is still in need of much work.

Progress

In the past 5 to 10 years a great deal of interest has been generated in matters related to women's health. Advocacy groups and members of Congress have requested more research into the causes, treatment, and prevention of diseases that affect the health of women. Major governmental agencies such as the National Institutes of Health, the Food and Drug Administration, and Department of Agriculture have responded to numerous congressional inquires regarding the lack of attention to women's health. Current efforts are being made to further the study of the health of women.

In 1990, the National Institutes of Health (NIH), a federal agency charged with the extension of a healthy life and reduction of illness and disability for all Americans through scientific research created the "Office of Research on Women's Health." NIH and other institutions are working to understand sex differences in the incidence and death rates from disease. This should lead to improvements in prevention, treatment, and health care for women.

More Is Needed

Although strides are being made to improve research pertaining to women, a recent Gallup Organization survey sponsored by the North American Menopause Society found that barely one third of women's sources of menopause information came from their physicians, and of those who did receive information, many felt that physicians failed to address their primary concerns. The majority of women were relying on the general news media such as magazines, books, journals, television, newspapers, or friends. Clearly, these are not always the most reliable source of accurate medical knowledge.[1] This book can help.

Chapter One
Dispelling the Myths

Many of the current attitudes about menopause have developed more from myth than from fact. Viewing menopause from an historical perspective helps to bring into focus our own feelings about the subject. Culture, medical trends, and most especially the family experience influence how a woman gains insight into this process. Being aware of our individual feelings and understanding the origins of these feelings are the first steps to opening ourselves up to new information and new ideas. Let's review some of the stories and stereotypes that exist.

MYTHS

Psychological Experience
History strongly suggests that menopause is a psychological experience or response. This usually derives from a woman's own self-perception, her current role in society, her present activities, and undoubtedly from her mother's menopausal experience. When information about an event comes from emotional perceptions, the response to that event is bound to be emotional. Individuals bear this out. For instance, a woman who perceives her mother as having had difficulty with menopause may fear that her future holds a similar experience for her. If a woman was raised to believe that menopause signifies the onset of old age, she may fear a loss of personal attractiveness and/or fear that she is no longer

7

useful in society. A woman who has devoted her entire adult life to the role of mother is especially susceptible to depression as she perceives this role to be ending. In fact, any woman who normally has difficulty dealing with other life transitions may have difficulty during the menopause transition. Finally, a woman experiencing problematic menstrual periods could easily assume that menopause will be one more difficult hurdle that she must conquer.

These sad stereotypes need not exist if emotional perceptions are replaced with facts. Although some women experience sadness over loss of reproductive capabilities, relief from the physical discomforts of monthly bleeding, painful periods or dysmenorrhea, premenstrual tension, possible pregnancy, and contraception is a welcome alternative. In addition, for those who do experience some problems, measures now exist that can ease the burden.

Culture

A woman's culture strongly dictates her response to menopause. Some cultures promote a positive outlook.[1] For example:

- The women of Newfoundland are well informed and outspoken about this stage in their lives.

- Among the Mandurucu of South America, menopause is perceived as a graduation from the more subservient role of the female to that of male status as the oldest woman maintains authority over the entire family, which may number more than 50.

- In East Africa, the older women assume many political and social leadership roles.

- Mayan Indians of Mexico welcome menopause because it raises them to a new status personified by acceptance and respect as an elder. They not only are released from childbearing concerns, but are relieved of household chores which are delegated to the wives of married sons.

- Japanese women maintain their self-image by refusing to consider themselves menopausal.

In cultures where menopause and aging are viewed negatively, the response of the woman differs significantly.

- In Ghana where the postmenopausal wife may be replaced by younger wives, these postmenopausal women frequently believe themselves to be witches.

- Not long ago in Ireland, the belief held that no role existed for women who had completed their reproductive lives.

Although the influence of culture persists, the impact of current medical research should dispel many of the myths that abound.

Evolution Of Medicine And Menopausal Thinking

Menopause has not always been viewed as a normal developmental change in a woman's life like puberty has. Some of the early medical thought on menopause proposed a connection between menopause and chronic disease or long-term disease. Others called it a "time of trial, often of suffering and danger."[1] Many psychoanalytical writers have typically regarded menopause as a critical event that was a threat to the adjustment and self-concept of middle-aged women. Deutsch, in 1945, referred to loss of reproductive life as a partial death.[2] In 1963, a physician by the name of Wilson described menopause "as a strange endogenous misery...the world appears as though through a gray veil and they live as docile, harmless creatures, missing most of life's values."[1] Even as late as 1970, "Menopause from the Psychiatrist's Point of View" stated that "an assumption had been proposed that women's ability to work reduces to a quarter of the normal by menopause."[1]

For years medical research on menopause was nearly unheard of and physicians usually worked only with women who experienced problems during menopause, so their experience justifiably taught them that menopause was a negative event. Adding this to society's view that menopause was a topic not to be discussed created many dilemmas for women. No wonder many women responded to the menopause with various complaints of illness. Preparing for the event was unheard of and merely discussing it was thought to be most inappropriate. No effort was made to encourage mothers and daughters to foster discussions since menopause was regarded as a "taboo" topic.

Hormones Made Me Do It!

As knowledge of how the body worked progressed, medical researchers discovered hormones and their link to the female body. Instead of putting to rest many of the myths existing about feminine behavior, hormones became the excuse. The influence of hormones on female behavior has received considerable attention for some time. The premenstrual syndrome with its "raging hormones" received blame for any unusual change in a woman's behavior. Believers in a relationship between hormones and behavior have come to believe this interaction ultimately affects women's decision-making abilities; thus, the role of women in "responsible" positions has been questioned! To complicate attitudes toward women's behavior even more so, some of the more positive aspects of a woman's psychological response to life, e.g., caring, sensitivity, thoughtfulness, which have been described as positive aspects in the work place could be used against her. For example, a woman in an administrative position who made special concessions for a good employee with a short-term problem, was blamed for being too lenient, compromising, and lacking a "get tough" attitude. Likewise, if of menopausal age, a woman's outbreak of emotional behavior could be attributed to the menopause; it made little difference if the outburst may have been justified.

Men And Hormones

Consider that men's behavior is rarely judged in terms of hormones although they too can have varying degrees of mood swings and vacillate in their decision-making processes. They seem to rarely if ever receive the extent of negative criticism that a female does. Men experience declining hormone levels during their lifetimes. The difference between men and women is that women's changes in hormonal status are more abrupt than are those of men.

"Male Menopause" Middle-aged men can suffer from the loss of sexual prowess causing much psychological discomfort and this can be a critical threat to their virility and masculinity. Sexual response time may diminish along with the ability to achieve and maintain erections. Men may compensate for these threats through divorce, extramarital affairs, purchasing flamboyant sports cars, and changing hair styles to correct thinning hair. Strangely enough, society is more willing to accept these erratic and often detrimental actions than to accept the menopausal woman's mood swings and changes in temperament.

Menopause Stereotype
"No Longer A Woman" A normal sequence of events conspired to create the stereotype of the typical woman experiencing menopause. As discussed earlier, recent history defined menopause as marking the end of a woman's womanliness. Supposedly with the loss of her "good looks," other major changes occurred in her life that contributed to a psychological instability. With children raised and usually gone, not only did the woman feel lost, but also ambivalent or confused about her current role. A woman often found that she and her spouse had drifted apart while he advanced his career and she devoted herself to the children. This woman easily became depressed, experienced a number of psychosomatic complaints, and developed a number of other problems one of which could have been a dependency upon alcohol to "pick herself up." To some degree, it was almost an expected behavior. The common stereotype of the menopausal female was that of a woman with multiple complaints who found comfort in the physician's office.[1] Unfortunately physi-

cians only saw menopausal women with complaints since the healthy menopausal female had no reason to seek the advice of the physician. Thus physicians understandably developed a negative view of the menopause experience.

Work Place The typical stereotype of the woman experiencing menopause has used the "stay-at-home-mom" as the norm. Nearly 50% of the work force today is made up of women and this necessitates a study of the positive and negative aspects associated with being a member of the career world during menopause.

The work place provides a different set of factors that have their own impact on the menopause scenario. A career outside the home serves to minimize menopausal discomforts as work offers a distraction. Women in the work place seem to have less difficulty coping with some of the menopause transition happenings than their counterparts who remain at home.

However, the work place can become a "double-edged sword." Hot flashes during working hours can create embarrassment and discomfort when clothes become damp and dishevelled and makeup becomes streaked and "cakey." Moreover, long-term sleep deprivation due to the same hot flashes can contribute to anxiety, irritability, and an inability to think clearly, creating "frazzled nerves" which may lead to conflicts with colleagues and others. Knowledge and planning can alleviate many of these problems.

Single Woman The single state, whether by divorce, death, or preference, bears its own set of problems. Although many of the same concerns affect married women, the impact may be more severe for a single woman since she may not have the financial backup or support systems.

For single women, the cessation of childbearing capability may bring forth a buried subconscious awareness that it "really is too late for childbearing." The chances of being a "natural mother" are over. Career-wise, menopause may signal that a woman has not achieved what she had hoped for and time is running out. Success in the work place is critical for most single women, since society seems to have a negative image of the aging woman in the work place, contrary to the male image, whose position seems to improve with age. In our society, many men avoid the stumbling block of age, as they are perceived as more knowledgeable and more attractive as the aging process occurs. No such buffer exists for the aging female.

As the sole support for herself and perhaps of her children, anxiety can take hold. Is her job stable? Is it too late to change careers? Is it too late to try something new and different? Has she planned adequately for her retirement?

Menopause Does Not Occur In A Closet

Fact and fiction interweave to create myths. Understanding menopause entails unravelling its myth to expose the fact. The menopausal woman is not an "hysterical female," but often during this time many life crises can occur to create the image of a woman "out-of-control." During these years

- a woman's aging parents may need various types of care
- a woman may lose a spouse or his economic contribution to the family through illness
- friends may be lost through death or disability
- children who have left home return with multiple problems of their own
- retirement may be looming on the horizon and financial security may be at stake

Menopause shares a relationship with these events. A problem develops when the response that results from these crises is interpreted to be due to the menopause while the real problem remains unnoticed. It seems that both the health care professional and the menopausal woman can confuse the issues and not deal with the real problem.

Know The Real Problem

Many women approaching or in the midst of the menopause transition period are very concerned with changes that are occurring to their bodies and the lack of control that some of these changes seem to impose. Although an inevitable part of a woman's life, it is not one that should be taken lightly. Quite the contrary! Women move through this period with a wide variety and intensity of symptoms. Some women will experience more symptoms while others will have few or no reactions. Poor communication can lead to inadequate or improper treatment. A better sense of awareness by health professionals and women can lead to appropriate solutions.

Menopause As A Transition

Menopause is a transition, and with all transitions the potential for crisis exists, but an equal potential for unparalleled opportunities for growth also exist.[3] One's attitudes and skills can make the difference.

REALITY

Present Concerns

To start looking beyond the menopause fiction, overviews of two current health issues, cardiovascular disease and osteoporosis, are presented. This book covers each topic with associated treatments in greater detail later.

Overview

The lack of the ovarian hormone estrogen seems to be a major contributing factor in the postmenopausal diseases of osteoporosis and cardiovascular disease, two of the leading causes of illness and death in older women. Although some controversy exists over whether this is due to aging or decreased hormones, a number of studies have shown that a deficiency of estrogen has a very definite effect.[1]

Cardiovascular Disease Cardiovascular disease (CVD), disorders of the heart and circulatory system, is the leading cause of death for both older men and WOMEN. Most people picture an elderly overweight man as the likely candidate for a heart attack, yet heart disease is the number one killer of American women, accounting for approximately 50% of all deaths in women over the age of 50. During the childbearing years, estrogen protects women against CVD even when women have the same risk factors for heart disease as men, such as smoking, high blood pressure, and elevated cholesterol levels. However, the protection is only temporary, and each year after menopause the risk increases. The picture is not as glum as it may appear, however, since CVD can be prevented, or the severity decreased with early recognition, proper diet, exercise, and the use of estrogen.[4]

Osteoporosis Osteoporosis is another very important health issue for middle-aged women, and is best described as a loss of bone mass which results in thin, brittle bones. Although osteoporosis affects aging men and women, the impact is seen most dramatically in the white female following the menopause. African-American women attain a greater bone mass and are therefore less likely to experience osteoporosis. The relationship of osteoporosis to menopausal status, more so than to chronological age, is demonstrated best in a study that evaluated the bone mass of 50-year-old women who had their ovaries removed 20 years earlier compared with those of 70-year-old women who had gone through a normal menopause 20 years earlier. The bone loss for both groups was comparable and nicely illustrates the influence of estrogen on maintenance of bone mass.

The most common sites of bone loss are the vertebrae (backbone or spine), the hip, and the radius (wrist), all of which are subject to fractures. Vertebral or spine fractures result in curvature of the spine or "dowager's hump," and falls are usually the cause for hip and wrist fractures.

Prevention is the key factor. A number of studies have shown a relationship between maintenance of bone mass and estrogen therapy. Exercise and calcium, alone and in combination with estrogen also have a positive effect on bone.

DEBUNKING THE MYTH

Recent research shows that in reality menopausal women as a group do not utilize health care services anymore than would be expected considering the increases in age.[5] In addition, the Massachusetts Women's Health Study, the largest and most comprehensive, prospective, longitudinal, long-term study of middle-aged women to date, reported "menopause, as a natural event, that appears to have no major impact on health or health behavior." Further it states that "the majority of women barely notice the menopause," and provides a powerful argument that the menopause period is not and should not be viewed as a negative experience.[6]

Studies such as these reinforce the notion that menopause is a normal stage of development or a normal physiological event, and that most of the symptoms and problems of the middle-aged woman may be due to social and personal events in life or other factors rather than the changes associated with the menopause period.

The question of whether menopause is a normal event or a disease is really not important. What is important is that treatment is available for the symptoms and consequences of menopause. Short-term symptoms of menopause might include hot flashes and urinary tract and sexual problems; long-term consequences include osteoporosis and cardiovascular disease.[7] The most important and currently controversial method of treatment today for these symptoms and consequences is hormone replacement therapy. Much more information on this topic will be offered later in this book.

PAST AND PRESENT

For too long, many myths surrounded the menopausal period of a woman's life. The increase in the numbers of the aging population has prompted a good deal more interest in this topic. Consider that life expectancy for the female in 1900 was approximately 50 years, and the average age for meno-pause was reported to be 51 years. Menopause was simply accepted as a part of the aging process; and since many women never lived long enough to experience it, menopause was not a problem! This average has not changed for the woman of the 1990s; fifty-one is still the average age women experience menopause today. But some things have changed. Two centuries ago, less than 30% of women lived long enough to reach menopause; currently, 90% do, including more than 30 million American women with an average post-menopausal life expectancy of 28 years.[8] Today the average woman can expect to live another 30 years beyond meno-pause. Thus it becomes apparent and important to know how to live out the second half of life in the very best way, and there is no reason to believe that it should not be the "better half."

Chapter Two

Menopause—What is it?

L eaving behind what menopause is not, this chapter will
provide answers to what menopause is. In order to gain
a better understanding of the reaction of the female
body to decreasing hormone levels, it is helpful to know first,
how the different phases of this process are defined.

OVERVIEW

MENOPAUSE is simply a transition from the reproductive to
the nonreproductive state. Menopause means the last period—officially declared with Follicular-Stimulating Hormone
(FSH) levels greater than 40 mIU per mL and one year of no
periods. The date can be accurately pinpointed except this
accuracy can only be achieved "after the fact." The entire
sequence of events progressing to menopause can start for a
woman in her 20s or 30s when estrogen production begins to
taper off.

Not long ago, menopause was considered a short-term
physiologic event in a woman's life. Now the medical community realizes the shortsightedness of this idea since the
effects of estrogen deficiency that begin prior to menopause
are lifelong and diverse. While all women experience menopause as the end result of a decline in estrogen production,
not all women will experience the same symptoms that
accompany this decline. At the end of this chapter, an explanation of the symptoms that may occur will be provided.
Planning for the menopause transition and all the years fol-

lowing entails long-term preparation. With care this transition period can and should be the very best time of your life!

DEFINITIONS

In order to gain a better understanding of the reaction of the female body to decreasing hormone levels, it is helpful to know that the process is divided into several phases. The names and definitions of each phase are provided below.

Menopause ("Change of Life") is said, by most, to have occurred when no menstrual period has taken place for 12 months (in the absence of pregnancy) and to signal the end of fertility or the reproductive years.

Premenopause is the period of active ovarian estrogen production.

Postmenopause is the period of time following actual menopause and when little or no estrogen is produced by the ovaries.

Perimenopause refers to the time immediately before and after the menopause.

Climacteric defines the time span in which the ovaries gradually decrease their production of estrogen. This time period begins during the years prior to menopause and ends during the postmenopausal years.

Little disagreement exists over the definitions of menopause and pre- and postmenopause, but confusion does arise over the sometimes interchangeable use of the terms perimenopause and climacteric.

WHEN WILL THIS HAPPEN?

A decrease in hormones can be responsible for hot flashes which may occur as early as five years to ten years prior to cessation of menstruation. The climacteric may span from age 35 to 50 or longer. The average age of menopause is 51.4 years, with an average range of 45 to 55 years. Although it has been suggested that the age of menopause might be increasing, numerous sources of information indicate that it has remained fairly constant for centuries. When menopause occurs at 40 years of age or younger, it is classified as premature menopause.

MENSTRUAL CYCLE AND HORMONES

In order to fully appreciate what happens to your body as it ages, a description of how menstruation occurs is in order and will help you better understand why the body acts the way it does.

The menstrual cycle cannot be understood without an explanation of the hormones involved. Estrogen, a hormone closely linked to menstruation and menopause, has already been mentioned. Other important hormones will be named throughout this chapter.

Hormones are chemicals produced in special glands in the body. They travel through the bloodstream carrying important messages to other parts of the body. Once a hormone reaches its destination, the message it carries causes a specific change to occur.[1] Each hormone carries its own message and causes distinct reactions in the body. The notion of how hormones work need not be complex; it is merely a cause-and-effect relationship. Glands produce hormones which cause an effect somewhere else in the body. The overview of the menstrual cycle explains how hormones function in this process.

Ovaries And Eggs

As mentioned earlier, the ovary is the female reproductive gland that produces the female egg. The ovary may also be called a female gonad. Women naturally have two ovaries found to the right and left of the uterus. See Figures 2-1 and 2-2.

The normal menstrual cycle is the result of a complex set of interactions between the ovaries, the female reproductive glands located deep in the pelvic region of the body, and the pituitary gland located at the base of the brain. Other glands and hormones are also involved in this process, but the ovary

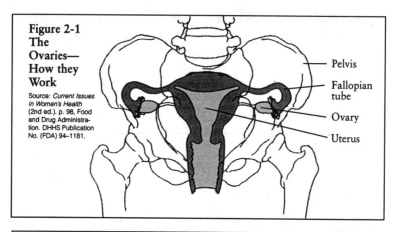

Figure 2-1 The Ovaries— How they Work

Source: *Current Issues in Women's Health* (2nd ed.). p. 98, Food and Drug Administration. DHHS Publication No. (FDA) 94–1181.

Pelvis

Fallopian tube

Ovary

Uterus

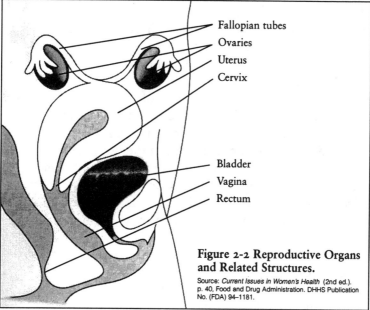

Fallopian tubes

Ovaries

Uterus

Cervix

Bladder

Vagina

Rectum

Figure 2-2 Reproductive Organs and Related Structures.

Source: *Current Issues in Women's Health* (2nd ed.). p. 40, Food and Drug Administration. DHHS Publication No. (FDA) 94–1181.

and pituitary glands play major roles in the two phases of menstruation: the follicular phase and the luteal phase.

The ovaries contain structures called follicles that hold the egg cells. The follicles are important to hormone production. Females are born with egg cells which number approximately 1 to 2 million and by puberty only between 200,000 and

400,000 remain. The degeneration process allows only a few hundred or thousand of egg cells to survive by the time of menopause. Only about 500 eggs will mature through ovulation where the eggs actually leave the ovary. These eggs are either fertilized by a sperm, or if not fertilized, expelled during the menstrual period.

During puberty the female hormones estrogen and progesterone stimulate the reproductive system to mature and cause menstruation to begin.

The Brain

Two glands are found near the brain that affect the menstrual process: the pituitary gland and the hypothalamus. The pituitary gland is connected to the brain and produces hormones that regulate growth and activity of other glands. The hypothalamus, located in the brain regulates many basic body functions and plays a role in the production of hot flashes.

Both the pituitary and hypothalamus play a part in the beginning of the follicular phase of the menstrual cycle. The accompanying drawing (Figure 2-3) will help to explain the following descriptions of hormonal activity during the menstrual cycle.

Follicular Phase

Hypothalamus   The hypothalamus produces gonadotropin-releasing hormone (GnRH) which acts on the pituitary gland to release the gonadotropin-follicle-stimulating hormone (FSH) and luteinizing hormone(LH). FSH stimulates the development of follicles in the ovary. The follicles are sacs that hold the eggs and produce estrogen.

Follicle   One follicle becomes dominant, increasing its estrogen production to help the egg mature. In response to estrogen, the endometrium (lining of the uterus or womb) thickens. If pregnancy does not occur, this lining will be shed as menstrual bleeding. Estrogen also circulates to the pituitary and causes a midcycle surge of LH.

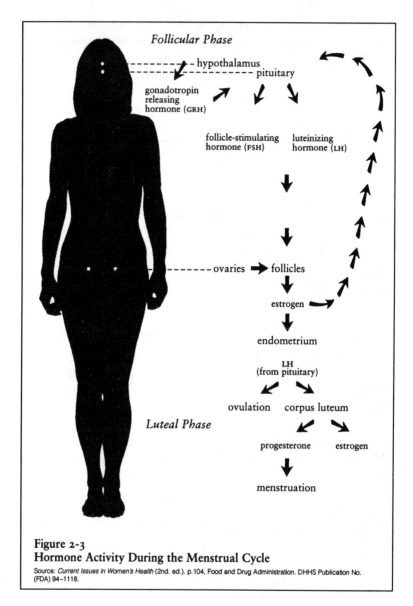

Figure 2-3
Hormone Activity During the Menstrual Cycle
Source: *Current Issues in Women's Health* (2nd. ed.). p.104, Food and Drug Administration. DHHS Publication No. (FDA) 94–1118.

Ovulation During ovulation the follicle ruptures and releases the mature egg. Under the influence of LH, the ruptured follicle is transformed into the corpus luteum. At this point two events can occur, either the egg is fertilized and the body prepares itself for pregnancy, or the egg remains unfertilized and menstruation begins. If pregnancy occurs, the corpus luteum is needed to maintain pregnancy. The luteal phase now begins.

Luteal Phase

Fertilization In the luteal phase, the corpus luteum produces both estrogen and progesterone. The progesterone makes the lining of the womb more receptive to the fertilized egg. Progesterone also prevents the pituitary from releasing any more gonadotropins and halts further follicular growth.

No Fertilization If fertilization does not occur, the corpus luteum disintegrates, estrogen and progesterone levels drop, and the thickened lining of the uterus is shed during menstruation. The entire process then begins all over again.

More Hormones

The physiological processes that occur in a woman's body— the menstrual cycle, pregnancy, menopause—are complex. Medical research attempts to define this complexity through studies. Because of their importance, estrogen and progesterone are the focus of many of these investigations. Further information is provided on the production of estrogen and progesterone in this section. Three new terms will be introduced: **estradiol, estrone,** and **androgen.**

Estradiol Recall that gonadotropin-releasing hormone (GnRH) stimulates release of follicle-stimulating hormone (FSH) which acts on the ovarian follicle to promote maturation of the egg. The ovarian follicle produces the most potent estrogen, the sex steroid, estradiol. Although the ovary is not the only site of estradiol production, almost 90% originates there.

GnRH also stimulates release of luteinizing hormone (LH) which in turn causes the release of the egg and the formation of the corpus luteum. The corpus luteum produces estradiol which is released into the blood to be circulated throughout the body. Estradiol and progesterone are released into the blood to be circulated to their receptor sites where they effect other parts of the body.[2]

Estrone   Estrone, another form of estrogen, is produced through two routes. The first route involves glands, such as the adrenal glands located near the kidneys. The adrenal glands produce estrone directly. The second route deals with the conversion of other hormones, such as testosterone, to estrone. Estrone accounts for about 10% of estrogen production prior to menopause—after menopause, is the primary estrogen produced in the body.

Androgens   Androgens are the source of all steroidal estrogens in the bodies of men and women. Androgens are vital to the production of estrogen outside of the ovary. This production occurs by means of a conversion process called the "peripheral conversion" process which takes place in body fat and to a lesser degree in brain, bone, and other sites, including possibly muscle tissue.[3] Two androgens key to estrogen production are **androstenedione** and **testosterone.**

The primary source of androstenedione and testosterone is the ovary before degeneration of the ovarian follicle. Following ovarian follicle degeneration the adrenal glands become the most important production site of androstenedione and testosterone, with androstenedione as the primary product as shown in Figure 2-4. The conversion of androstenedione to estrone, and testosterone to estradiol occurs mostly in body fat, and to a lesser degree in the brain, bones, and other sites. Androstenedione also converts to estradiol, but estrone is the primary product. As if this versatility were not enough, androstenedione may also convert to testosterone.

Progesterone   Progesterone is another sex steroid produced by the corpus luteum and released into the bloodstream to affect other parts of the body.[2]

Hormone activity is complex, but a familiarity with the hormones will aid understanding of their effects on the body

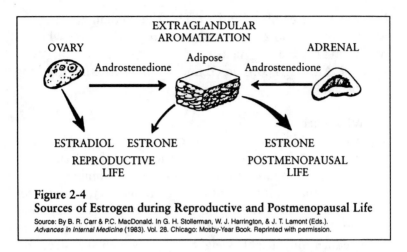

Figure 2-4
Sources of Estrogen during Reproductive and Postmenopausal Life
Source: By B. R. Carr & P.C. MacDonald. In G. H. Stollerman, W. J. Harrington, & J. T. Lamont (Eds.).
Advances in Internal Medicine (1983). Vol. 28. Chicago: Mosby-Year Book. Reprinted with permission.

and current treatment methods which will be discussed later in this book.

It is important to understand the effects of hormones on the body. Furthermore the measurement of hormone levels provides an indication of processes that are occurring within the body and the stages these processes have reached. For example, a gradual elevation of FSH levels may provide the first indication of menopause. Significant FSH elevations are particularly diagnostic of menopause. Blood and urine samples are used to monitor hormone levels.

CYCLE LENGTH

With the exception of pregnancy, the monthly cycle repeats over more than 30 years of a woman's life. During the early stages of menstruation, the average cycle length is 29 days. This cycle length decreases slowly but steadily with time. At 20 years of age, it is about 28 days, and by age 40 it may have dropped to about a 26 day cycle.[4]

WHEN IS "IT" OVER?

Age
Most women in the United States will experience menopause

between the ages of 45 and 55 with the median age at 51.3. Some women stop menstruating as early as age 35, whereas others may continue menstruating until age 55 OR EVEN LONGER. Although considered normal, menstruating this long is unusual.

Why Then?

The age at which menopause occurs is genetically predetermined, unlike the age of menstruation, which is related to body mass. Menopause has no relation to the number of prior ovulations, that is, it is not affected by pregnancy, breast feeding, use of oral contraceptives, or failure to ovulate spontaneously. It is also not related to race, socioeconomic conditions, education, height, weight, age at which menstruation began, or age at the last pregnancy.[5] Many of these factors have been implicated at some point in time in the menopause picture, but conclusions are difficult to draw because facts are either limited or lacking. One newly discovered factor though is smoking. Recent studies have found that smokers experience menopause earlier than nonsmokers by about 2 years.

A Gradual Process

Menopause does not happen abruptly unless it is caused by a hysterectomy with surgical removal of the ovaries. It is a gradual process in which the levels of estrogen and progesterone slowly decrease over a number of years. As the number of follicles in the ovaries decrease, hormone production slows, and the transition from regular ovulatory cycles to cessation of menstruation is characterized by a change in cycle length and bleeding patterns. Even after menopause, women's bodies continue to produce estrogen, but far less of the hormone is made in the ovaries. In postmenopausal women, a majority of circulating estrogen is produced through the conversion process in which the adrenal gland makes hormones (androstenedione and testosterone) that will be converted by stored fat or the liver to estrogen. However, far less estrogen is produced in this manner than is produced in the ovaries before menopause.

Conversion Levels

The greater the amount of body fat present, the greater the amount of conversion of androstenedione to estrone. For this reason obese women are less likely to develop symptoms of estrogen deficiency and are less likely to develop osteoporosis. Therefore, the greater the amount of body fat, the better the opportunity for continued estrogen. However, as is well known, excess weight may lead to other far more serious problems. For example, in some women enough estrone is produced by conversion to cause growth of the lining of the uterus, even to the point of excessive growth causing bleeding which may be indicative of uterine cancer. Therefore, a woman who is overweight and has stopped menstruating and starts bleeding/menstruating again should be examined by her health professional to determine the cause of the bleeding. On the other hand, a slim body is a risk factor for both osteoporosis and hot flushes/flashes.

THE PROCESS

In some women, menstrual periods continue to occur at regular intervals until they stop abruptly and permanently. Usually the change is more gradual. Over a period of 1 to 3 years, the amount of bleeding decreases, the interval between bleeding episodes lengthens, and periods in which there is no bleeding increase in duration. Final menstrual periods may be represented by only slight spotting. This change in bleeding pattern occurs because of a progressive decline in ovarian estrogen secretion. Bleeding ceases permanently when too little estrogen is being produced to cause growth of the inner lining of the uterus.

On the other hand, some women have increased bleeding before the menopause. Bleeding episodes may occur as often as every 2 to 3 weeks and may be prolonged and profuse. This may be due to erratic increases and decreases in estrogen secretion. Any changes in the normal menstrual pattern should always be investigated by a health professional.

For most women, menopause is usually a gradual and

smooth process with minimal problems. Although menopause signals major changes, it definitely should not require a change in life or lifestyle. Some women experience uncomfortable side effects such as hot flashes, night sweats, and vaginal changes all as a result of estrogen deficiency. However, estrogen deficiency can cause far more serious long-term related problems such as osteoporosis and heart disease which will be discussed in later chapters.

HOW CAN I BE CERTAIN

Usually if you have not had a menstrual period for a year, you can be reasonably certain that you have reached menopause. Further confirmation can be accomplished by a blood test to determine your level of follicle-stimulating hormone (FSH). Levels above 40mIU/mL prove you have reached menopause.

Surgical Menopause

Premenopausal women who have their ovaries and uterus removed surgically experience many of the same signs and symptoms as those women who experience menopause naturally, however surgical menopause can be quite different. If both ovaries and uterus are removed, menopause will take place abruptly, and the hot flashes and vaginal and urinary tract symptoms will occur soon after surgery. These hot flashes may be more severe, more frequent, and last longer. Hormone replacement therapy with not only estrogen, but sometimes androgens is in order for these women since natural testosterone levels also fall dramatically after the ovaries have been removed.

If only the uterus is removed (hysterectomy), a surgical menopause does not occur since the ovaries are left intact. Menstruation will stop, but the symptoms of menopause will not be experienced. Some women who have a hysterectomy without removal of the ovaries may experience menopausal symptoms at a younger age. This is thought to be due to decreased blood supply to the ovaries secondary to surgery.

Surgery Trends   Prior to the 1970s, it was common to remove ovaries along with the uterus since it was believed that this was one way to prevent ovarian cancer. However, it has been found that women who have both ovaries and uterus removed are at higher risk for osteoporosis and cardiovascular disease due to changes in estrogen and lipid levels and bone metabolism. Current recommended practice now is to leave the ovaries intact in the premenopausal women unless there is a clear reason to remove them.

Most hysterectomies, regardless of age, are performed for removal of uterine fibroids. Other common reasons for removal of the uterus include endometriosis, uterine prolapse, cancer, and abnormal uterine bleeding. The average age for hysterectomies is about 42 to 43 years of age, an age which has been fairly consistent over the years.

WHAT TO EXPECT

All women who survive to midlife will experience menopause,however their experiences will not all be the same. Menopause maybe a "nonevent" for many women who encounter few if any symptoms, while other women may experience troublesome physical and emotional difficulties such that they seek professional help. Many of the common symptoms are described here, but remember a woman need not experience any of them.

Hot Flashes

Hot flashes are one of the more common and earlier signs of menopause occurring in 75-85% of pre- and postmenopausal women in the United States. For years it was thought these hot flashes were "all in the head." No one could ever have drawn this conclusion after having witnessed a woman in the process of a hot flash! It was not until about 1975 that hot flashes were studied intensely and found to have a definite physiological cause.

Cause Of Hot Flashes Hot flashes appear to be caused by a decrease in the estrogen levels, affecting the hypothalamus in the brain. Since the hypothalamus also regulates body temperature, the disruption of hormonal balance at menopause can cause a "mistake" in temperature control. Measurable events occur during the hot flash; skin temperature rises significantly and blood flow and heart rate increase. During the hot flash, the face and neck become bright red due to the localized dilation of the blood vessels. The body attempts to compensate for the increase in temperature much like it does with a fever. The blood vessels of the skin enlarge to allow for heat loss through the skin and sweating occurs which also causes a loss of heat.

Frequency And Sensations Hot flashes can occur off and on before other signs of menopause are evident. Among women who do have hot flashes, the pattern and form may differ. Some begin to have hot flashes when menstrual periods become irregular, others well before the menopause, when menstrual periods are still regular.

Many women report some kind of a warning prior to the onset of the hot flash such as a tingling sensation, pressure in the head, or anxiety which is distinctly separate from the hot flash and may last from 5 to 60 seconds.

Hot flashes can best be described as a feeling of intense heat that usually starts on the head, neck, chest, and upper body that increases rapidly and lasts from a few seconds to several minutes. They may be accompanied by anxiety, palpitations, dizziness, headache, or nausea. Profuse sweating, enough to saturate the clothing, follows while the body attempts to readjust and cool. The frequency, intensity, and duration of the individual hot flash episode vary among and within individuals. For some women, hot flashes can occur as often as several times a day to two or three times a week, and for some less frequently or not at all. Most women have them infrequently, but approximately 10 to 15% have recurrent and severe hot flashes. The period of time over which hot flashes are experienced is 6 months to 2 years, although there are some women who report hot flashes for 10, 20, or more years. Although hot flashes can occur without any obvious cause, some women have found that precipitating factors may be stress, emotions, a confining space, spicy foods, alcohol, and caffeine.[6] External temperature has also been found to have an effect on hot flashes; there is a significant reduction in both the frequency and intensity of hot flashes in a cooler environment.

Night Sweats   The hot flash that occurs during the night is called a night sweat and can bring as much, if not more discomfort than hot flashes that occur during the day. Night sweats interfere with sleep which may lead to insomnia resulting in chronic fatigue, irritability, and depression. Some authorities believe that these symptoms are due to estrogen depletion, but there is lack of agreement in this area. It does make sense that if a woman is awakened several times during sleep on an almost nightly basis drenching in sweat, having to get up and change her nightclothes and bedding followed by subsequent inability to fall back to sleep, then chronic fatigue, irritability, and depression would follow! Although hot flashes and night sweats can be disruptive to a woman's daily activities, they are not dangerous in and of themselves. In most cases hot flashes are not severe and usually disappear after a few months. It is uncommon for a woman to have hot flashes that last more than 5 years after menopause.

Who Is At Risk?   Why some women experience hot flashes and others do not is not clearly understood. Neither age when menstruation begins nor the number of pregnancies seem to have an influence. However it has been found that obese individuals are less likely to develop hot flashes, because they do not have as great a decrease in estrogen levels due to the presence of fat.

As stated earlier, during and following menopause the ovaries and the adrenal glands produce androgens, androstenedione, and testosterone. In postmenopausal women androstenedione is converted to estrone (a form of estrogen) in body fat, and the rate of conversion increases as individuals age. With a greater amount of body fat, more estrone is produced. For this reason, obese women are less likely to develop symptoms of estrogen deficiency.

MANAGEMENT OF HOT FLASHES

Estrogen Therapies

Hormone replacement therapy (HRT), principally estrogen, is currently the most effective treatment for hot flashes. Many studies have proven this over and over. A representative study conducted in the early 1970s used one group of women who were treated with estrogen and the other group who were "treated" with a placebo (a pill without estrogen, sometimes called a "sugar pill"). The women on estrogen reported a dramatic decrease in their symptoms; but when they discontinued treatment, their hot flashes returned. When the group who was taking the placebo started on estrogen, their hot flashes disappeared. The women were unaware of which type of pill they were receiving—placebo or estrogen.

Estrogen Estrogen for hot flashes can be administered either by mouth or by a skin patch. The skin patch is called a transdermal estradiol skin patch. If control of hot flashes is the primary goal of treatment, the lowest dose that will control the hot flashes is used.

Progestins Progestins [medroxyprogesterone acetate (MPA)], a form of the hormone progesterone, have been used in the treatment of hot flashes when estrogen therapy has failed or in women who do not want to take estrogen. However, the dose that may alleviate hot flashes may be a higher dose than is normally used, and may have a negative effect on cholesterol levels. Many times those women who cannot take estrogen cannot take progestins either. Hence, the following recommendations may prove helpful.

Nonestrogenic Therapies

Although estrogen has traditionally been the drug of choice for relief of hot flashes, drugs without estrogen, or nonestrogenic drugs, are available and can alleviate hot flashes to some degree. Women who cannot take estrogen or dislike the side effects and who may not be helped by estrogen, are likely candidates for nonestrogenic therapy. Some of the more common nonestrogenic therapies are described below.

Oral Androgens (testosterone)   Oral androgens or testosterone are used effectively in the treatment of hot flashes, night sweats, depression, and disturbances of libido. They do not prevent vaginal problems, or coronary artery disease, and are probably ineffective in preventing osteoporosis. Oral androgens are most effective when combined with estrogen.

Bellergal   (phenobarbital, ergotamine, and belladonna alkaloids) Bellergal relieves some symptoms such as hot flashes, night sweats, restlessness, and insomnia, but has sedative effects and is not considered a treatment of choice. Also bellergal can be habit-forming.

Clonidine (an antihypertensive drug)   Clonidine relieves hot flashes. Side effects include severe episodes of low blood pressure, insomnia, dizziness, nasal stuffiness and mood swings.

Vitamin E   Some studies and "off-the-record" reports have shown a decrease in hot flashes with the use of vitamin E. Most studies failed to indicate how much to take, how long it should be taken, and who should take it. Additional study is required to determine the true effect of vitamin E on hot flashes.

Tranquilizers   Tranquilizers relieve some depression and restlessness, but are not good substitutes for estrogen replacement. They do not relieve hot flashes.

Nonmedicinal Therapies

Temperature   Control external temperature if possible, for example sleep in a cool room. When temperature cannot be controlled, wear layered or lightweight clothing. Avoid polyester and synthetics if at all possible.

Self-awareness   Know when to expect hot flashes and the triggers which cause them.

Behavioral therapies   Taking part in stress reduction strategies and relaxation techniques to decrease the frequency of hot flashes may be helpful.

Smoking   Decrease, or better yet, stop smoking. Evidence of decreased estrogen levels in smokers would indicate that smoking may increase the risk of hot flashes.

Acupuncture   Early information shows a decrease in frequency of hot flashes with the use of acupuncture, but the information is not yet adequate to make any kind of recommendation.

Diet   Eliminate those foods which seem to "trigger" hot flashes such as those mentioned previously, e.g., hot drinks, spices, alcohol, etc. Keep your own food and activity diary to determine what aggravates and alleviates your hot flashes.

Exercise   Be active. Although further investigation is necessary in this area, scattered studies and informal evidence suggest a decrease in frequency and intensity of hot flashes among women who exercise regularly.

Herbal remedies   Use herbs and other natural medicinal substances cautiously. Some plants have estrogenic properties which should be avoided in those women in whom the use of estrogens is contraindicated. Ginseng is a perfect example, since it is a potent source of plant estrogen. When you are taking ginseng, you are still taking estrogen; it can affect your body the same way pills, patches, and creams affect your body. Even the lining of the uterus can thicken since no progesterone is being used to counteract the effect of the estrogen.[7]

BEHAVIOR CHANGES

Stereotype

Mood and behavior changes have been associated with the menstrual cycle since ancient times. Psychiatric syndromes have been associated with depression following childbirth, premenstrual syndrome, hysterectomy, and menopause. Historically both physicians and menopausal women have blamed a number of psychological symptoms on the menopausal transition period. More recent advances in the study of this transitional period have negated this logic which assumed that since the two events occurred at the same time one must be the cause of the other. The picture of the raging or depressed menopausal woman with frequent mood swings is a myth. Much of the information that supported this myth was based on poor, flawed, or outdated studies.

Even some of the more recent research suggests a need for additional study in the area. A study of women aged 50 to 59 on estrogen therapy showed evidence of depression; whereas, untreated women of the same age did not. After age 60 the reverse was true, the treated were not depressed and the untreated were. The lack of depression in those over 60 may have meant that long-term estrogen therapy with associated decreases in hot flashes and relief from physical discomforts works.[8]

PMS, Menstrual, Pregnancy Blues

Mood fluctuation studies have found that women during the premenstrual and menstrual weeks (when estrogen levels are low) reported a greater incidence of negative moods and conditions such as depression, tension, irritability, restlessness, anxiety, migraine headaches, sleep disturbance, and impaired concentration. Whereas, during the midcycle (when estrogen levels are higher), patients reported feelings of well-being and elation. Notably during the final trimester of pregnancy when the impact of both social and physical impediments are felt, depression is uncommon probably due to high and stable levels of estrogen. However, during the weeks following delivery when estrogen levels are low, postnatal depression is common.

In contrast, there are those who have found that in the years preceding menopause when estrogen levels fluctuate, psychological symptoms are more apparent and seem to subside or disappear in the postmenopausal years when estrogen levels, though low, are stable. Providing estrogen replacement therapy therefore appears to be logical during these difficult times.[9]

Estrogen And The Brain

During the last twenty years, many studies have failed to show a consistently higher rate of depression in postmenopausal women.[1,10,11] Hence, wide disagreement exists regarding depression, increased nervousness, anxiety, insomnia, and headaches and their relationship to decreased estrogen levels. It does seem appropriate, however, to add the dimension of the role of estrogen and its influence on brain chemistry. As referred to earlier, estrogen receptors in the brain play a part in the expression of hot flashes. Likewise, it has been found that estrogen influences the level of serotonin in the brain, which when decreased, is thought to be an important factor in depression.

Life Stressors

Clearly a number of changes occur in a woman's life at about the same time as the menopause transition period takes place. Children usually leave home at about this time, divorce may create a need to seek employment. For the employed woman, limited career advancement or opportunities may be apparent, a parent, spouse or other close relative may die, or the woman may begin to develop some physical illness herself. All people respond differently to stressors in their lives. Some become depressed while others overcome these same stressors by redirection in more positive ways like exercise, pursuing hobbies, or engaging in volunteer activities.

Most authoritative sources however support the notion that menopausal women are no more depressed than the general population. According to many studies, the cases of depression reported are more related to "midlife stressors" than to the menopause.

Perspective

To put all of this in perspective requires insight into the fact that psychological symptoms in menopausal women are neither universal nor inevitable. Several groups of women have been studied who have shown little or no psychological symptoms during the menopause transition. It cannot be overlooked, though, that a majority of menopausal women who do seek medical attention have prominent psychological symptoms, some of which seem to respond to hormone replacement therapy.[12,13,14]

MEMORY

Although memory impairment is a common symptom noted by many women in the menopausal transition phase, very little is actually known about this phenomenon. Memory impairment is thought to be related to decreased estrogen levels, however, the few studies that have evaluated the effect of hormone replacement therapy on cognitive function have shown contradictory and inconsistent results. These conflicting results are believed to be due to poor test design.

Some studies are worth mention. Women who experienced surgical menopause and were given estrogen replacement were found to have better memory and abstract reasoning scores than their counterparts who were given placebos instead of estrogen.[11]

But results of a 15 year study conducted in California on 800 women with an average age of 76 years found no consistent evidence to indicate that estrogen preserved memory function in old age.[12,13] More attention is being paid to this area, and many women are reporting that their memory is improved with the use of estrogen; but many of the reports are being dismissed as hearsay. Clearly more evidence is required to justify the use of estrogens for the maintenance of memory function in postmenopausal women.

SLEEP DISTURBANCE

Hot Flashes

Hot flashes at night (night sweats) clearly contribute to disrupted sleep. The pattern that develops could be considered a "domino effect": night sweats to sleep disruption to insomnia to irritability and fatigue in the daytime.

Depression

Depression also contributes to poor sleep, and decreased estrogen levels allegedly affect mood which can result in depression.

Research

Some of the research on sleep disorders in postmenopausal women have attributed sleep problems to decreases in rapid eye movement (REM) sleep and increases in the sleep-latency level. Both are thought to be due to low estrogen levels. One study demonstrated that individuals who took estrogen noticed improved sleep and felt refreshed upon awakening as compared with the group who did not receive estrogen.

Although sleep disturbance in menopausal groups seems to be an expected event, most of the research that has been conducted thus far seems to indicate that the menopausal status itself may play a minor role, with the exception of night sweats which can clearly be linked to decreased estrogen levels. Changes in lifestyle and more awareness and concern over physical problems may be of greater significance in sleep disturbances.[15]

Simple Remedies

The good news is that since sleep problems are not all necessarily related to decreased estrogen levels, measures other than estrogen replacement therapy, may be used to help relieve them.

In the absence of any serious sleep disturbances or conditions which contribute to these disturbances, some very simple remedies may help the habitually poor sleeper.

- Arise at the same early hour daily irrespective of how much sleep you may have had during the night. Stay on this schedule, even on weekends, to acquire a consistent sleep rhythm.

- Go to bed at approximately the same time nightly.

- Do not use your bed for anything but sleep. No television or reading. Sexual activity is the exception.

- Exercise vigorously for approximately a half hour daily but not before bedtime.

- Perform relaxation exercises at bedtime.

- Eliminate caffeine sources which include coffee, tea, colas, chocolate bars, and the sinful hot fudge sundae! Sometimes as few as two cola drinks or cups of coffee in the afternoon can affect sleep.

- Eliminate alcohol and nicotine. Alcohol does cause relaxation, but as it wears off, one often awakens and is unable to fall back to sleep. Other research studies have shown that nicotine in smokers causes an increased alertness.

- Avoid excitement prior to bedtime in the form of television, reading materials or stressful interaction with others.

- Take a warm bath prior to bedtime to relax.

- Have a warm drink or a light snack prior to bedtime. Avoid heavy meals close to bedtime.

If any of these measures do not help resolve the insomnia problem, then further investigation by a health professional is in order. Furthermore, avoid the use of over-the-counter sleeping products unless recommended by a health professional. Many of these products contain antihistamines which can cause fatigue and depression the "morning after."

Drowsiness may lead to daytime napping which further disrupts restful sleep patterns causing more of a need for the "sleeping pill."

REPRODUCTIVE ORGAN CHANGES

The outstanding physical changes in the reproductive organs after the menopause are directly related to the loss of estrogen.

Labia

The pink (usually found in women with fair complexion, may range from dark to even black in Asian/Mid-Eastern and African-American women) folds of skin in the pubic region are called the labia majora and labia minora. A decrease in estrogen causes physical changes to this area. Much of the labia is fat tissue,and fat is gradually reabsorbed. The labia minora, the small folds situated between the labia majora and the vaginal opening, may actually disappear. Thinning of the pubic hair also occurs.

Vagina

The vagina, which has the highest concentration of estrogen receptors in the body, gradually narrows, and the vaginal walls become thin and dry, and lose their elasticity. Sexual intercourse may be painful, and vaginal irritation may occur. Lack of vaginal lubrication from a decrease in the production of vaginal secretions may contribute to the problem. A vaginitis (infection or inflammation of the vagina) may develop causing itching, burning, discomfort, painful intercourse, and vaginal bleeding.

Support Structures

All body organs are held in place by supporting tissues, usually muscle or ligaments. The supporting structures of the uterus, bladder, and rectum lose much of their tone and strength because of shrinkage in the tissues themselves. These changes in supporting structures and the weakness in the vaginal wall may result in the uterus "dropping" and pushing on the vagina. A portion of the bladder or intestines may push into the vaginal wall which leads to a feeling of heaviness, or as described by some women "feels like my insides are dropping."

The use of estrogen, either by mouth or skin patch, or by way of the vagina with suppositories, creams, or tablets, will reverse the thinning of the vagina and will help alleviate many of the associated problems.

Vulvar Irritation or Vaginitis

The decrease in estrogen production which may promote a thinning of the vaginal wall may also change the acidic conditions in the vagina and allow the growth of problem-causing bacteria. Many postmenopausal women experience vaginal itching and discharge. The condition may range from annoying to debilitating. Antibiotics and antifungal drugs, either oral or vaginal, do not always eliminate the problem; antibiotics can sometimes cause a problem or make the problem worse. Estrogen therapy will thicken the vaginal lining, decrease vaginal dryness, and increase the acidity of the vagina, usually resulting in elimination of the problem. Other ways to control vaginal itching and discomfort include:

- Use of oatmeal or cornstarch baths
- Avoid the use of perfumed soaps, deodorant spray, and prepackaged cleansing tissues.
- Wipe from the front to the back after urinating or after a bowel movement.
- Check your sugar intake; sometimes a diet high in sugar encourages fungal infections. Repeated infection may be a sign of diabetes, so consult your health professional.
- Try a moisturizing gel called Replens® or Gyne Moistrin®; sold over the counter to counteract dryness and the irritation due to a lack of estrogen, and to raise the acidity of the vagina and prevent infection and inflammation.

URINARY INCONTINENCE

What Is It?

Many women believe that with age an inability to control urine flow eventually develops. An inability to "hold" urine is known as urinary incontinence. Not everyone will experience this problem. The advertising world would have you believe the opposite, because billions of dollars of incontinence management products are sold each year by them. The solution to urinary incontinence is not in covering up the problem, but in finding the cause and identifying the appropriate treatment. Urinary incontinence can occur most anytime in a woman's lifetime, or it may never occur. Menopause and advancing age increase the likelihood of developing the problem.

The lower urinary tract includes the bladder, a sac that holds the urine; the urethra, a tube that carries urine from the bladder to the outside; and the muscles in the pelvic area. Estrogen is needed to keep the urinary tract tissues healthy. These structures shrink as estrogen levels in the body begin to decline. This shrinkage accounts for the troublesome problems with urination such as leaking of urine when coughing, sneezing, or laughing; inability to hold urine resulting in embarrassing accidents; a more frequent desire to urinate; burning on urination; and an increased incidence of cystitis (bladder infection) or other urinary tract infections.

Treatment

Health professionals should be consulted before a woman embarks on a "self-treatment" regime, since infection may be present and will usually not go away without treatment. Other correctable problems may also exist, so see your medical specialist.

Estrogen replacement therapy can often correct urinary tract changes and symptoms. Estriol, a naturally occurring weak estrogen, may also be used.

Strengthening Exercises

Practicing simple exercises is encouraged to improve bladder function. Kegel exercises work the pelvic muscles and can be performed several times a day. Perform this exercise by squeezing or contracting the muscles in the pelvic area where the vagina and bladder openings are located. The best way to learn is while urinating; start the urine stream, then stop the flow by squeezing the muscles together. Once the squeezing and relaxing motion is learned, this exercise can be done while sitting, standing, or lying in bed. Even if weakened by the loss of estrogen, tightening and relaxing this muscle 20 to 30 times a day causes a significant improvement or cure.

SEXUAL FUNCTION

Changing Desires

During and after menopause, interest in sex may increase, decrease, or stay the same. Many factors including menopause can contribute to changing desires. Women should be aware of the factors that influence them and not just blame menopause or old age.

Both males and females show a decrease in total sexual activity or outlet with aging according to Kinsey and others.[16] The total sexual outlets per week in married females is approximately two per week for women in their twenties; this gradually decreases to once every other week for women in the sixties.

Good Attitude

Women who have had an enjoyable sex life prior to menopause are likely to keep the same attitude after menopause. Freedom from fear of pregnancy, discarded birth control devices, and finally the privacy and freedom from interruption can make sexual relations more enjoyable than they may have ever been. Some women may experience some change in sexual function during the years immediately before and after the menopause.

Life Influences

While changes in hormone production are usually cited as the major reason for lack of interest in sexual activity, other factors unrelated to hormone levels may come into play. For example, some women who have had a disinterest in sex for many years may use the menopause as an excuse to stop having intercourse. The question often asked is "Is declining interest in sexual activity the cause or the result of less frequent sexual relations?" Common sexual complaints include loss of desire, decreased frequency of sexual activity, painful intercourse, diminished sexual responsiveness, and dysfunctions of the male partner. Women who think that menopause and aging lead to the loss of femininity may lose interest in sex.

Helpful Strategies

At any age, sexual problems can arise if there are concerns regarding performance. If both partners are informed about the changes that occur during the aging process and communication regarding some of the related problems is open and candid, a successful sex life can be achieved well into the 70s and 80s and even beyond!

- For those women who experience pain during intercourse, estrogen replacement therapy in the form of pills, patches, and vaginal creams will improve the integrity of the vaginal lining and can make intercourse comfortable again. Most women notice improvement within a few weeks.

- Having intercourse on a regular basis may help improve lubrication, keep vaginal muscles toned, and preserve the size and shape of the vagina.

- Extending foreplay prior to intercourse will allow sufficient time for the natural secretions to lubricate the vagina.

- For those individuals who cannot take estrogen, or choose not to, nonprescription products such as K-Y jelly, Lubrin® or Replens® can relieve vaginal dryness and irritation; also enhances sexual enjoyment for those women taking estrogen therapy.

- Sitz baths can relax muscles and stimulate vaginal secretions.

- For infections, medical treatment is required. Estrogen may restore the thin vaginal and bladder tissues and lower the risk of infection.

- Testosterone levels also play a role in sexual motivation. During the reproductive phase of a woman's life, the ovary produces approximately 25% of the circulating testosterone. In the postmenopausal woman who has had a natural menopause, testosterone levels are considerably lower than those of younger women. The addition of testosterone to an estrogen replacement regime has been found to enhance sexual desire and increase interest and enjoyment of sex in the postmenopausal woman.[17]

- Despite the physiological changes that occur as a result of menopause, the most important factor in vaginal health is continued sexual activity and the presence of a functioning desired male.

- Some women live normal, complete lives without the "need" for sexual outlet in spite of the fact that there is nothing in the biology of aging that shuts down sexual function. It is not that they have "turned sex off," but the absence of a functioning, desirable male is not always uppermost in their minds. They still enjoy many aspects of life, remain psychologically healthy, and pursue a number of interests. Vaginal health can still be maintained with the use of estrogen therapy; and for those who prefer or cannot take estrogen, the use of vaginal lubricants such as Gyne-Moistrin® or Replens® may be helpful.

SKIN

The skin is a protective, supportive structure. Changes in the skin have a direct relationship to the loss of estrogen in menopause. As estrogen diminishes, the skin becomes dry and shrinks; collagen, the supportive structure, also declines. Thickness tends to decrease at the rate of 1% per year and collagen at the rate of 2% per year in early menopause.[16] The skin collagen content declines at a greater rate during the early post menopausal years as opposed to the later ones. If treated with hormone replacement therapy, much of this loss can be prevented or possibly reversed. However, while HRT may help, don't look for a complete rejuvenation.[18,19,20,21]

WEIGHT GAIN AND MENOPAUSE

Obesity is a major health problem in the United States and is particularly troublesome and problematic for women. On average, adult American women, as they age, show an increase in body weight. This overweight trend increases with age until 55 to 64 years, then begins to level off. Increased risk for high blood pressure, diabetes, and high blood cholesterol are associated with an overweight condition. Overweight is also an independent risk factor for heart disease.[22]

Research
The 1988-91 National Health and Nutrition Examination Survey (NHANES III) showed an increase in overweight among women ages 20 to 74. NHANES II, conducted from 1976–1980, showed a 27% increase where NHANES III demonstrated a 35% increase. NHANES III also showed a higher overweight rate among African-American and Mexican-American women as compared to white women.[22] Many women claimed this weight increase began around the time of their menopause.

Body Fat Distribution
Even more important than overall body fat is the distribution of body fat. Two body fat distribution types are recognized: the upper-body or abdominal fat distribution often called the "apple-shaped" body or male-type distribution of fat tissue and the lower body or hip fat referred to as the "pear-shaped body" or female-type distribution. Abdominal type fat distribution is more strongly associated with cardiovascular heart disease and death than is fat distributed around the hips. This abdominal or truncal fat, as it is often called, is associated with increases in low-density lipids (LDL), decreases in high-

density lipids (HDL),and an increased risk of coronary artery disease and death. A 12 year study of women in Sweden found degree of abdominal fat to be a strong predictor of heart attack.[23]

Effects Of Body Fat Distribution   There is general agreement that body composition in women changes with age, and these changes, independent of weight gain, have been found to begin around the time of menopause and continue to progress. Some of the general effects are the following:

- Total body fat percentage increases in relation to total body weight which may be explained by an estrogen-deficient state. Prior to the menopause, there seems to be no increase in fat mass in body composition.

- Adipose or fatty tissue increases mainly over the trunk and in the intra-abdominal area.

- The loss of fat-free body mass fat or increase in body fat is thought to be partly responsible for a decrease in resting metabolic rate (RMR). The RMR is the minimum amount of energy used to maintain our body functions. It is slightly higher than the well-known basal metabolic rate. What this means is that less energy is required to maintain bodily functions.

Diet And Exercise

Dietary and/or exercise interventions have been found to offset these changes in energy metabolism, body composition, and body fat distribution.[24] Exercise and an increase in lean body mass are responsible for increasing the resting metabolic rate. Continuous participation in aerobic activities such as walking, cycling, aerobic dancing, and swimming during the menopause transition and beyond will reduce and prevent the accumulation of body fat, especially in the upper truncal regions, thus lowering the risk for cardiovascular disorders.[25,26]

What all of this means is that we must exercise more, sit and eat less, which is what women have known for years, and now there is scientific evidence to support it! It is just that it is difficult to accept, and even more difficult to change old habits. But it is never too late to start!

CONCLUSION

Menopause brings a variety of sensations and experiences—some pleasant, some not so pleasant. Many of the perturbing episodes can now be managed as the medical field continues to investigate the mechanisms and hormones involved in the menopause process.

Chapter Three

Osteoporosis

One of the most critical health problems facing American women today is osteoporosis: a disease causing bones to become thin, fragile, and highly prone to fracture. Although not solely a woman's disease, 80% of the more than 25 million Americans affected by this condition are women. Characterized by back pain, loss of height, spinal deformity, and multiple fractures, osteoporosis produces fear—a fear that one possibly casual movement may result in a fracture or fractures producing pain, loss of movement, and loss of independence. Statistics demonstrate that one in every two women over the age of 50 will suffer a fracture resulting from osteoporosis.

FRACTURES

Osteoporosis develops gradually and, like high blood pressure, is a well established condition before it becomes apparent. This slow development is one of the reasons why it is often called the "silent epidemic." The disease is often well under way before symptoms are evident so treatment cannot cure, only manage the disease. Osteoporosis may not be noticed until a fracture occurs. Actions that would normally cause no problems in the average person can lead to a broken bone for a person with osteoporosis. Any bone in the body may be affected, but the hip, wrist, and spine or vertebrae are the most common sites of injury as shown in Figure 3-1.

Hip
According to the National Osteoporosis Foundation, the chance of a woman developing a potentially life threatening

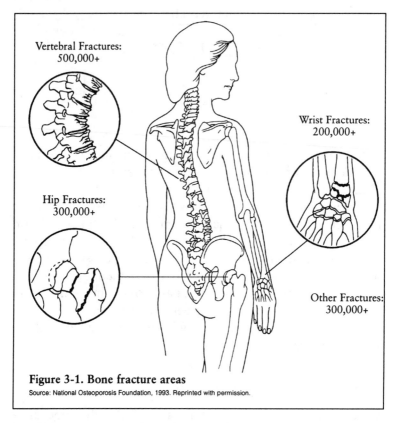

Figure 3-1. Bone fracture areas

Source: National Osteoporosis Foundation, 1993. Reprinted with permission.

hip fracture is equal to her combined risk of developing breast, uterine, and ovarian cancer. A hip fracture is the most serious consequence of osteoporosis as reflected in the following information:

- the frequency of hip fractures for women over age 75 is twice that of men; between 5 and 20% of people die after a hip fracture;
- postoperative complications of hip fracture include blood clots and pneumonia;
- between 12 and 20% of those who suffer a hip fracture do not survive the six months following the fracture;
- nearly half of the survivors require help in performing daily living activities;

Hip Fracture Patients | *Among more than 250,000 hip fractures annually*

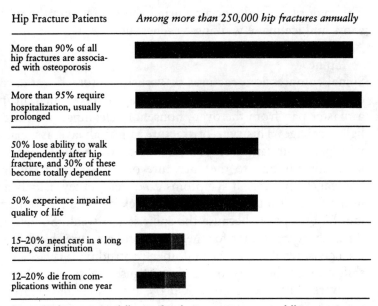

More than 90% of all hip fractures are associaed with osteoporosis	
More than 95% require hospitalization, usually prolonged	
50% lose ability to walk Independently after hip fracture, and 30% of these become totally dependent	
50% experience impaired quality of life	
15–20% need care in a long term, care institution	
12–20% die from complications within one year	

Note: Within one year following hip fracture, a person may fall into two or more categories

Figure 3-2. Effects of hip fractures

Source: National Osteoporosis Foundation, 1992. Reprinted with permission.

- 15 to 20% of those who suffer hip fractures lose their ability to function independently and require nearly one year of long-term institutional care; and

- only a small percentage recover completely. Figure 3-2 demonstrates this information.

Wrist

The likelihood of suffering a hip fracture increases with age; whereas, fractures of the wrist occur more frequently prior to age 75. Wrist fractures increase in number around menopause and level off after age 65, probably because of the rapid loss of bone in the years immediately following menopause. Wrist fractures occur in women who are relatively healthy and active and have good reflexes. Extending an arm to break a fall, causing the hand and forearm to bear the weight of the fall, is the usual cause of a wrist fracture.

The majority of falls occur during the winter months when snow and ice make walking treacherous.

Spine

Spinal compression fractures or "crush fractures" can develop from such simple actions as bending to make a bed, lifting a roaster pan from the oven, household cleaning, or lifting a light package. This type of fracture is not always associated with pain, but can be responsible for decreased height as one ages, contributing to the curvature of the spine or familiar "dowager's hump." If symptoms do develop, they usually are in the form of muscle spasms. The back muscles try to maintain body support because the spine is too weak. Sometimes the body compensates for these vertebral fractures by shifting the pelvis, resulting in the abdomen protruding forward. This shift crowds the intestines and can cause digestive problems. A severe shift may even crowd the lungs making breathing difficult. Stooped posture and loss of height not only changes the way a person looks, but how one feels about oneself. This is yet another reason to take measures to prevent osteoporosis. See Figures 3-3 and 3-4.

Cost

In addition to the personal cost, osteoporosis also has a social cost. Altogether, over 1.5 million fractures resulting from osteoporosis occur annually at a cost of $10-12 billion, which may approach $18 billion when other costs such as lost earnings and other social costs are considered. By the year 2020, unless dramatic steps are taken in the prevention arena, costs are expected to grow to $60 billion as shown in Figure 3-5.[1]

Fracture Rates

Scandinavia ranks higher in fracture rate than the United States, but the United Kingdom rate falls below the United States. Information from other regions is limited, but fracture incidence is lower among whites of Hispanic origin and among Blacks. White women 60 years of age or older have at least twice the incidence of fractures as African-American women.

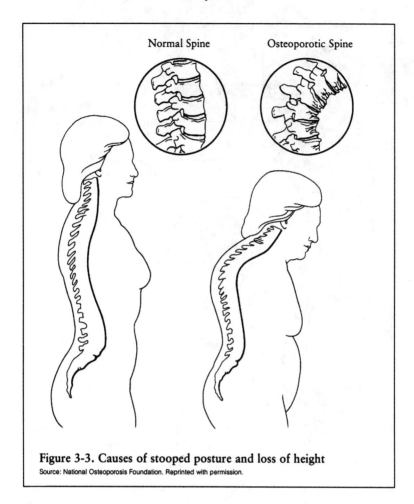

Figure 3-3. Causes of stooped posture and loss of height
Source: National Osteoporosis Foundation. Reprinted with permission.

Still, one out of five African American women are at risk of developing osteoporosis.[2]

Causes

A loss of estrogen can lead to the development of osteoporosis, but the menopausal condition alone cannot be blamed for the likelihood of developing this disease. Other lifelong factors such as calcium intake, exercise, cigarette smoking, alcohol consumption, caffeine intake, heredity, and race all contribute. Since lifelong actions can lead to the development of

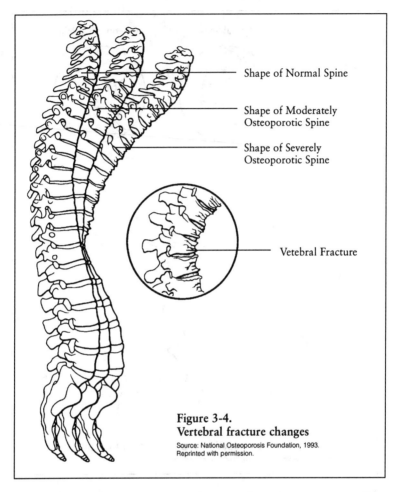

Shape of Normal Spine

Shape of Moderately
Osteoporotic Spine

Shape of Severely
Osteoporotic Spine

Vetebral Fracture

Figure 3-4.
Vertebral fracture changes
Source: National Osteoporosis Foundation, 1993.
Reprinted with permission.

osteoporosis, preventative measures must focus on altering
these habits. Before understanding all that is involved in the
development of osteoporosis or the disease itself, a discussion
about bone is necessary.

BONE

Bones comprise the strong bony frame that supports the body.
Although seemingly hard and lifeless, bone is a living, growing tissue. The fact that an infant develops an adult frame

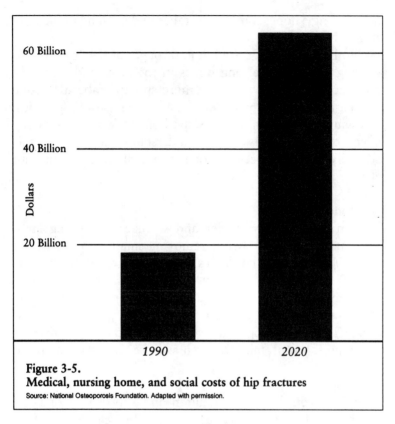

Figure 3-5.
Medical, nursing home, and social costs of hip fractures
Source: National Osteoporosis Foundation. Adapted with permission.

demonstrates this. Understanding that bone development changes with age is crucial to understanding osteoporosis.

A protein substance called collagen forms the initial structure of bone. The collagen framework hardens when calcium phosphate is deposited. Therefore, collagen and calcium work together to give bone its strength. The blood holds a small fraction of the body's store of calcium, the remainder resides in the bones and teeth of the body.

Bone Structure

Bone typically has two structures. The hard, dense, compact structure familiar to us is called cortical bone. Cortical bone forms the outer portion of bones and accounts for 80% of all bone. The second structure, referred to as trabecular bone, has a spongy, honeycomb appearance and is found in the interior of bone.

Both types of bone are found throughout the body, but to varying degrees. The long bones in the arms and legs hold more cortical bone, while the more spongy trabecular bone concentrates in the spine, pelvis, and the ends of long bones. Knowing the location of trabecular bone makes the damaging effects of osteoporosis easier to understand since osteoporosis critically affects trabecular bone, although cortical bone can also be affected.

Bone Growth

Human bones grow heavier and stronger by adding large amounts of new bone while removing small amounts of old bone. This process continues until approximately age 35. Growth then begins to slow and a reversal occurs, where withdrawal exceeds the addition of new bone. Several hormones and enzymes regulate this process, including testosterone in men, estrogen in women, calcitonin, parathyroid hormone, and vitamin D. Each will be discussed in more detail.

Rate Of Growth   The addition and subtraction of bone occurs at different rates throughout the life cycle. As an infant develops into an adolescent, bone growth is visible in the form of the child's developing frame. Although this growth rate begins to slow in adolescence, bone development continues until a "peak bone mass" or maximum density and strength of bone is reached. This peak bone mass is achieved between ages 25 and 35. A period of stability follows before bone loss begins.

The Critical Teen Years   The healthy development of bone cannot be emphasized enough when discussing osteoporosis. The development of bone begins in childhood, but the teen years are critical to achieving adult peak bone mass. During childhood and the teen years, new bone is added faster than old bone is removed. Recent studies show how important the teen years are to building bone. Women who drank a glass of milk or more per day up to age 25 showed significantly higher bone density in middle-age and older years than women who consumed less milk. Another study which followed teenagers for 11 years found a calcium intake of 800 to 1200 milligrams (mg) per day increased hip bone density when compared to lower calcium intakes. The health of bone in later years relies heavily on the preparation of bone in the childhood and teenage years.

"Pediatric Disease"   Past and present collide with osteoporosis—bone strength, determined by good dietary and exercise habits practiced in the early years of life, lays the groundwork for avoiding osteoporosis in later years. Osteoporosis has earned the title of "pediatric disease" because good bone formation in the early years plays a major part in prevention of the disease in later years.

Bone Loss

Two distinct phases of bone loss can be recognized: a slow, age-related phase that occurs in both sexes, and an accelerated phase which occurs in postmenopausal women. The slow phase begins around age 35 and continues into old age. Both sexes lose bone mass with aging, although men seldom develop signs or symptoms of osteoporosis before age 70. Men also can experience bone loss through decreased production of the male hormone, testosterone. This situation increases the risk of developing osteoporosis.

Women, because of their make-up, tend to be more susceptible to osteoporosis than men. At maturity, women typically have 10 to 25% less bone mass than men who achieve greater bone mass. In women, bone loss is further compounded by the process of menopause.

Premenopausal women over 30 years of age may lose less than one percent of their bone tissue annually, whereas these figures may reach three to five percent yearly during the first five to ten years following cessation of menstrual periods (postmenopausal period).[3] The most rapid decline of bone mass after menopause results in a loss of disproportionately more trabecular than cortical bone, making early prevention a top priority. Bone density continues to decline, and by age 85, more than 30% of the bone mass that one had at age 50 is lost. See Figure 3-6.

WHAT CAUSES OSTEOPOROSIS?

What do we now know about bone? Bone is continually building and breaking down at the same time. During the formative years, bone builds at a faster rate than the breakdown of bone occurs. Upon reaching a peak bone mass, this process levels off and reverses. At this stage, around age 35, the breakdown of bone begins to exceed the formation of bone. The less dense, spongy trabecular bone is more sensitive to bone loss than the compact cortical bone. The cortical bone is found in greater proportion on the outer skeletal parts such as the hip and long bones in the body. Loss of cortical bone occurs at a much slower rate, so osteoporotic fractures of the hip do not usually begin to occur until about age 70 or 75.

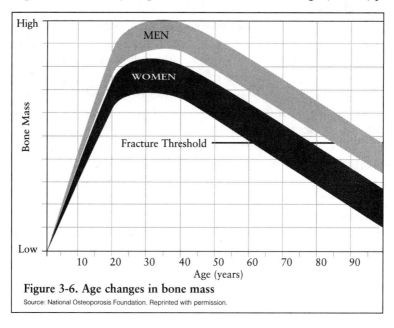

Figure 3-6. Age changes in bone mass

Source: National Osteoporosis Foundation. Reprinted with permission.

Vertebral bone (spine or backbone) is comprised primarily of trabecular bone and is known to be more susceptible to osteoporotic bone loss. That is why the beginning stages of a "dowager's hump and/or loss of height are seen more frequently in the early postmenopausal woman. Menopause can hasten this natural bone loss process leading to the development of osteoporosis. See Figure 3-7.

Calcium

A discussion of bones is not complete without considering the relationship of calcium to the bone growth process. Calcium supplies strength to bone, yet it has other crucial functions throughout the body. The blood allows free calcium to circulate throughout the human system. If the blood level of calcium drops below required levels and nutritional intake does not supply adequate replacement, calcium is taken from the bones for release into the bloodstream. Bone is weakened at the expense of other body functions.

The reverse also holds true. If blood calcium levels are high, the excess calcium can be deposited in bone. Hence, bone serves as a reservoir, storing nearly 99% of the body's calcium. The role of adequate nutritional calcium intake is evident in maintaining the balance between bone and blood

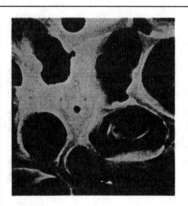 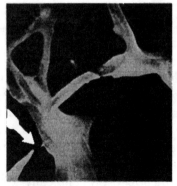

Figure 3-7.
Micrographs of biopsy specimens of normal and osteoporotic bone.
Source: National Osteoporosis Foundation, From Dempster, et al. Reprinted with permission.

calcium levels. Poor nutrition and low bone calcium reserves can be factors in the development of osteoporosis.

During the early 40s after "peak bone mass" is attained, calcium begins to leave bones faster than it is replaced, and bones become less dense or strong. This natural and gradual process that occurs in both men and women accounts for lifetime losses of calcium that range from 20% to 30% for males and up to 45% to 50% for some females. Bone loss in women increases approximately three to five percent per year beginning at the menopause transition and continuing for five to ten years thereafter. The body further compounds this problem by partially losing its ability to absorb calcium, which occurs at about age 45 in women and 60 in men.

Clearly, several complex factors influence the quality and quantity of bone, especially after the age of 40. These include:

- the amount of peak bone mass attained
- rates of bone loss due to menopause and aging
- calcitonin, a hormone produced naturally in the body and involved in calcium regulation
- calcitriol, an active form of vitamin D
- parathyroid hormone
- diet, especially calcium intake
- intestinal and kidney function
- physical forces that impact on bone such as body weight and exercise

Though bone loss occurs in most postmenopausal women, not all develop the degree of osteoporosis that results in fractures. Two predictors include 1) the amount of bone mass at the time of menopause and 2) the rate of bone loss following menopause. Current information also points to two strong contributing factors: a drop in estrogen levels in women due to menopause (technically known as "estrogen deficiency") and a chronically low intake of calcium ("calcium deficiency"). Together estrogen and calcium play an important role in helping bones stay strong.

WHO IS AT GREATEST RISK?

A number of risk factors for osteoporosis have been identified. The evidence for some of these factors is greater for some than for others. These include:

Age
Since bone loss in both sexes continues until 80 to 90 years, of age, age itself is a significant factor. Rapid bone loss, often seen in osteoporosis, is NOT a normal part of aging.

Gender
Osteoporosis is more common in women than in men, presumably because women have less bone mass and because they lose bone more rapidly than men due to decreased estrogen production.

Early Menopause
A strong predictor for the development of osteoporosis, many experts define "early" menopause as menopause occurring before the age of 45. A significant amount of bone is lost during the first ten years following menopause. Thus, the number of years past menopause, not age, directly affects the strength of bones. For example, if two women experience menopause, one at age 50 and the other at age 55, the woman at 55 has an additional five years of estrogen production in her favor. Likewise, the woman who undergoes a hysterectomy at age 40 and receives no estrogen replacement will have an additional 10 and 15 years of estrogen deficiency as compared to these two women.

Premenopausal Estrogen Deficiency
Estrogen deficiency in the premenopausal may be caused by excessive exercise or eating disorders such as anorexia nervosa or bulimia.

Race
Caucasians and Asians are at higher risk than African-

Americans; incidence is about twice as high in White women as in Black women.

Nulliparity
A woman who has never completed a pregnancy beyond an abortion (spontaneous or elective)

Small-boned And/Or Underweight
Large-framed women are at decreased risk, since they have more bone mass. The majority of estrogen production in the postmenopausal woman results from conversion of adrenal androgen which occurs mostly in fat tissue. However, these facts cannot be interpreted as an argument for obesity. Likewise, thin, small-framed men are at greater risk for osteoporosis than men with larger body structure and body weight.

Family History Of Osteoporosis
Susceptibility to fractures may in part be hereditary.

Caffeine Intake
While a high intake of caffeine from foods such as coffee, colas, and chocolate promotes bone loss through loss of calcium in the urine, a recent study shows that coffee consumption does not adversely affect bone if at least a cup of milk per day is consumed.[4] However, excessive amounts of caffeine, in any form, should be avoided until more studies are conducted to determine safe levels.

High Intake Of Sodium
A high intake of sodium increases calcium loss through the urine. A moderate intake of 2400 mg is generally acceptable.

High Intake Of Phosphates
Some experts believe that those whose diets include a high intake of red meat, cola drinks, and certain processed foods are at greater risk for increased bone loss. The Recommended Daily Allowance (RDA) is 800 mg.

High Animal Protein Intake

A high intake of animal protein ranges from an excess of the equivalent of four ounces of meat per day, to a diet over the recommended intake that is almost exclusively protein. Calcium loss occurs through the urine. Average protein intake requirements can be found in Chapter 6.

Chronic Low Calcium Intake

Adequate calcium intake is needed throughout one's life to build and maintain bones.

Alcohol

According to the National Osteoporosis Foundation, regular consumption of as little as two to three ounces of alcohol daily may be damaging to bones in young and middle-aged men and women. Beware of a recent study which found social drinking increased bone density in both men and women. Alcohol is Not recommended as a preventive measure for osteoporosis since evidence on the negative side is more convincing.[5]

Cigarette Use

Tobacco smoke interferes with the liver's ability to metabolize estrogen. Menopause generally occurs earlier in heavy cigarette smokers.

Lack Of Physical Activity Or Sedentary Lifestyle

Any degree of inactivity places one at risk for osteoporosis since it causes bone loss.

Excessive Physical Activity

Excessive exercise which leads to cessation of menstrual periods in young women can lead to decreased bone mass and eventually osteoporosis.

Medications

Certain medications may contribute to the risk of developing osteoporosis.

Glucocorticoids Or Corticosteroids   Glucocorticoids or corticosteroids (not the type used by athletes to increase muscle mass) may be used in the treatment of Cushing's disease, rheumatoid arthritis, osteoarthritis, asthma, lupus erythematosus, inflammation and diseases of the eye, liver disease, pulmonary disease, psoriasis, ulcerative colitis, and Crohn's disease, leukemia and other cancers in association with chemotherapy. Glucocorticoids and corticosteroids can be found under various names such as

- cortisone
- hydrocortisone
- prednisone
- prednisolone
- triamcinolone
- dexamethasone and others

Bone loss increases with the strength of medication and the duration of use. Glucocorticoids decrease calcium absorption.

Thyroid Hormones   Thyroid hormones in excessive amounts can result in greater amounts of bone removal than bone formation. These drugs are used in the treatment of hypothyroidism and for thyroid nodules. A blood test can be performed to determine if the thyroid hormone level is too high.

Anticonvulsants   Anticonvulsants, such as phenytoin and barbiturates which are used mainly to prevent convulsions and some heart irregularities, may cause softening of the bones which in turn can lead to osteoporosis. Sometimes your health care provider can use an equally effective drug without the consequences of bone loss.

Antacids With Aluminum   Antacids with aluminum are used for stomach problems, but when taken in large amounts can lead to bone loss through increased loss of calcium in the urine. Antacids are not meant for extended use. If increased doses are necessary to control symptoms, seek consultation with a health care provider.

Methotrexate   Methotrexate is a drug used in the treatment of a number of different types of cancers and immune disorders, such as arthritis. This drug affects bone forming cells and may also have a negative effect on kidney function, leading to increased calcium loss in the urine.

Cyclosporine A Cyclosporine A is a type of drug which is used in organ transplants and for some diseases of the immune system. It has been reported to lead to bone loss if used over extended periods of time. Cyclosporine A is frequently used in combination with glucocorticoids.

Gonadotropin Releasing Hormone Analogues Gonadotropin Releasing Hormone Analogues, which are used in the treatment of endometriosis, have been associated with bone loss. If treatment is short-term, bone loss may be regained.

Heparin   Heparin is used to prevent blood clotting. Although the mechanism is not understood, it impairs both bone breakdown and formation. Aspirin, also used to prevent clotting, does not have the same effect on bone.

Cholestyramine   Cholestyramine controls cholesterol levels and has been found to affect the absorption of vitamin D which may lead to decreased calcium absorption.

Other Medications   Other medications indirectly affect the person with osteoporosis. Sedatives, muscle relaxants, and blood pressure drugs can cause dizziness, lightheadedness, or loss of balance, possibly causing a bone fracturing fall. Combining drugs can intensify the action of other drugs, including those that can be purchased over-the-counter. Alcohol, a drug itself, should be used with caution, since even small amounts can interact with medications and interfere with balance and coordination. Always consult a health care provider prior to taking drugs other than those recommended or prescribed.

OTHER CAUSES OF OSTEOPOROSIS

Not only drugs, but also certain diseases can speed bone loss. Certain diseases have been implicated in the formation of osteoporosis. Having one of these diseases does not mean you have or will develop osteoporosis, but it does mean you are at greater risk. Conditions affecting the development of osteoporosis are:

- diseases of the thyroid and parathyroid gland, kidney disease, and certain forms of cancer such as lymphoma, leukemia, multiple myeloma
- impaired ability of the intestine to absorb calcium caused by diseases of the small intestine, liver, or pancreas
- liver disease
- rheumatoid arthritis
- chronic pulmonary (lung) disease

Health professionals can evaluate whether you have one of these disorders or are taking one of these drugs and work with you to avoid osteoporosis.

WHAT SHOULD I DO?

The following guidelines will be useful if either you or someone you know may be taking medications that cause or contribute to bone loss or are afflicted with a condition which may speed the development of osteoporosis.

- Discuss with your health care provider whether you are at risk for osteoporosis.
- Arrange to have a bone density test to determine bone status.

- Discuss medication dose and duration consequences.
- Discuss medication alternatives.
- Discuss treatment if necessary.
- Take steps to preserve bone mass in collaboration with your health care provider.
- Avoid risks as described earlier.

Complete the following questions to determine your own personal risk for osteoporosis. The more times you answer "yes" the greater your risk.

Question	Yes	No
1. Do you have a small, thin frame, or are you Caucasian or Asian?	☐	☐
2. Do you have a family history of osteoporosis?	☐	☐
3. Are you a postmenopausal woman?	☐	☐
4. Have you had an early or surgically induced menopause?	☐	☐
5. Have you been taking excessive thyroid medication or high doses of cortisone-like drugs for asthma, arthritis, or cancer?	☐	☐
6. Is your diet low in dairy products and other sources of calcium?	☐	☐
7. Are you physically inactive?	☐	☐
8. Do you smoke cigarettes or drink in excess?	☐	☐

Figure 3-8. Osteoporosis: Can it happen to you?
Source: National Osteoporosis Foundation. Reprinted with permission.

Further information concerning medication use can be found in "Medication and Bone Loss" from the National Osteoporosis Foundation. See Resource section at the end of the book.

DIAGNOSIS OF OSTEOPOROSIS

Silent Disease

People with osteoporosis may show no symptoms until their bones become so thin that a sudden strain, bump, or fall causes a fracture with subsequent pain and possible immobility. This lack of symptoms has earned osteoporosis the title of the "silent disease."

X-ray
Because no definitive signs exist to discover its presence, osteoporosis may first be found on an x-ray taken for another purpose. A regular x-ray will only detect bone loss exceeding 20 to 40%. Unfortunately, by the time a person has lost this much bone, the risk of breakage is already present.

Other Tests
Other methods for determining bone mass and bone density exist. These measurements are safe, simple, painless tests that evaluate bone density at various body sites and for the most part use small amounts of radiation. Bone mass measurements can often be helpful in deciding whether to begin a prevention or treatment program, yet they are not currently recommended for every woman. Some of the problems with these measurements are their lack of availability, poor quality of the results, lack of ease of performance, and expense. The ideal measurement should be noninvasive (does not enter the body with needles or tubes), reasonably precise and accurate, relatively inexpensive, and safe (low radiation exposure). Each test should also be capable of predicting an individual's risk for osteoporosis as well as response to therapy.[6] If your health care provider decides to test you for osteoporosis, one of the following tests may be suggested.

Single-Photon Absorptiometry (SPA) SPA was the first commercially available technique for the noninvasive measurement of bone mineral density. It measures bone mineral content in the forearm, wrist, and heel which are composed mainly of cortical bone.

Dual-Photon Absorptiometry (DPA) Typically used to measure the total cortical and trabecular mineral content of the spine and hip, the DPA, while able to predict the risk of future fractures as well as the response to treatment, has largely been replaced by Dual-Energy X-ray Absorptiometry. Nevertheless, the information obtained by DPA can be quite useful in the management of individuals who have or are at risk for osteoporosis, and uses approximately one tenth of the radiation that results from a routine chest x-ray.

Dual-Energy X-ray Absorptiometry (DEXA) A more recently developed technique, DEXA is used to measure the amount of bone tissue of the spine, hip, wrist, heel and total body. DEXA has greater precision, can be completed in a shorter time, and exposes the patient to slightly lower levels of radiation than DPA

Quantitative Computed Tomography (QCT) Commonly known as a CAT scan, QCT is the only method that can measure the density of either the entire bone or only the trabecular portion. Usually the vertebrae (spine) is the site of measurement. QCT can be used to determine spinal fractures and to monitor response to aging, disease, or therapy.

Ultrasound The ultrasound is one of the newer noninvasive methods of bone mass assessment or measurement. The major advantages of this method over others is 1) the ability to measure not only bone quantity, but also bone quality, and 2) there is no radiation exposure. This technique measures ultrasound velocity at the knee cap or heel.

Radiographic Absorptiometry (RA) A noninvasive x-ray of the hand is sent to a laboratory where a computer analysis is performed to determine bone mineral density.

Biochemical Markers Of Bone Turnover These new blood and urine tests can determine how rapidly bone is being removed and to what extent it is replaced with new bone. With these tests, bone loss can be identified prior to changes in bone density studies. Early response to treatment can also be measured. Although these tests cannot diagnose osteoporosis they can identify "rapid losers". Only a bone mineral density test can determine a person's current bone mineral density, diagnose osteoporosis, or predict a person's risk for future fractures.

Vitamin D Receptor Gene A vitamin D receptor gene (VDR) responsible for helping the body to use vitamin D, which plays an important role in bone and calcium metabolism, has been associated with osteoporosis. Further research is needed to determine exactly how variations in this gene lead to low bone density.

ARE STRONG BONES ALONE THE ANSWER?

The study of bone density alone cannot adequately predict the risk of fractures. Many factors such as a predisposition for falling, lack of neuromuscular coordination, race, body structure, calcium intake, activity levels, alcohol consumption, and smoking history may alter a person's susceptibility to fractures. Together bone measurements and risk factors can predict more fully those individuals for whom osteoporosis poses a considerable risk.[7]

OSTEOPOROSIS TREATMENT

The Role Of Estrogen In Osteoporosis

Good News The good news is that osteoporosis is a preventable and treatable condition. Estrogen intervention in the form of estrogen-replacement therapy (ERT) or hormone-replacement therapy (HRT) is the best documented method for preventing osteoporosis in women. Replacement therapy (ERT or HRT) reduces bone resorption (bone breakdown), prevents postmenopausal bone loss, and reduces fracture risk by reversing the changes associated with estrogen withdrawal. Estrogen stabilizes bone density by preventing further loss and may act directly on the bone leading to increased bone mass. Also effective in the treatment of established osteoporosis, estrogens prevent further bone loss and fractures.[7] Increased bone density produces stronger bones and reduces fracture rates.

Length Of Treatment Many studies have found for estrogen to be most effective, it should be given during the first five to ten years immediately following menopause, since this is the time when bone loss is greatest. Estrogen benefits continue for as long as therapy is provided irrespective of duration of treatment. When therapy is withdrawn, a faster rate of bone loss occurs suggesting that long-term therapy is best. A greater rate of bone loss occurs if therapy is stopped completely. This loss is greater than the bone loss that occurs in those who never received therapy.

When To Start Previously there was some debate over the effectiveness of administration of estrogen to the elderly postmenopausal woman. However, clear evidence exists that treatment at any age is necessary in those women who are at greatest risk, since the incidence of hip fracture increases with advancing age and the consequences are costly both economically and physiologically.

What Kind Of Estrogen? All the current information available to date tells us that all estrogens, in appropriate doses, reduce bone loss whether taken by mouth or through the skin (transdermal). Recent information also seems to indicate that estrogens taken on a daily basis, may be slightly more effective in the prevention of bone loss.[8]

For women who have NOT had their uterus removed, progestin (a synthetic form of progesterone) is prescribed along with estrogen. This combined hormone replacement therapy (HRT) eliminates any increased risk of uterine cancer, and the addition of progestin does not negate the beneficial effect of estrogen on bone mass. Women without a uterus have no need for progestin.

Other Drugs

A limited number of drugs have been approved by the U.S. Food and Drug Administration for the prevention and treatment of osteoporosis. As previously discussed, one of the best known is estrogen, which will be covered in greater detail in Chapter 5.

Calcitonin Calcitonin is a hormone produced in the thyroid gland that regulates calcium and bone activities. It not only prevents bone loss, but also alleviates the pain of osteoporotic fractures. Salmon calcitonin has been approved by the FDA. Calcitonin is safe, but cannot be taken by mouth, because it is inactivated by stomach secretions. Therefore, calcitonin, when used, can be administered by injection or by nasal spray, a new method, which was recently approved by the FDA. Miacalcin® nasal spray, which is recommended for women who either refuse or cannot tolerate estrogens, or others for whom estrogens are contraindicated, now offers an additional FDA approved medication for the treatment of postmenopausal osteoporosis.[9]

Bisphosphonates These chemical compounds slow bone loss and may even increase bone mass. A number of bisphosphonates are under study for the treatment of osteoporosis. Etidronate, a drug previously approved for another type of bone disease known as Paget's disease, was recently approved by the FDA for osteoporosis treatment. Alendronate, another member of the bisphosphonate family was also recently approved. These two drugs offer new treatment options to millions of women combating this debilitating disease.

Other compounds are undergoing research and are in the investigational stages. According to the National Osteoporosis Foundation (NOF), a national voluntary health organization dedicated to reducing the widespread prevalence of osteoporosis, the general use of these therapies is not encouraged since some of them have not been approved by the FDA for the prevention and treatment of osteoporosis.

Sodium Fluoride Although it has been used for almost 30 years for the treatment of spinal osteoporosis, sodium fluoride still remains an experimental therapy. Sodium fluoride has value for established osteoporosis and is known to have an influence on bone growth. Its usage remains controversial since the increased bone mass seems to be more susceptible to fractures than normal bone mass, and there are many side effects.

Vitamin D (Calciferol)   Vitamin D is formed in the skin following exposure to ultraviolet light and can be found in fatty fish, eggs, liver, butter, and multivitamins. Published studies have not conclusively demonstrated the effectiveness of vitamin D in the treatment or prevention of osteoporosis, although it is known to increase calcium absorption in the stomach. Too much vitamin D can be harmful and high doses can even cause bone loss. The RDA is 200 international units (IU) for adults; most multivitamins contain 400 IU, and milk contains 100 IU. The elderly should take a multivitamin with 400 IU of vitamin D. More than 1000 IU per day is not recommended.

Anabolic Steroids   These are synthetic derivatives of testosterone which appear to stop bone loss and may increase bone formation. Although studies have shown improvement in bone mass, none have shown a reduction in fracture rate. They can also cause liver abnormalities, fluid retention, and masculinizing characteristics as well as adverse or negative effects on cholesterol levels which may lead to heart disease.

Parathyroid Hormone   Parathyroid hormone may have a beneficial effect on bone mass, but safety is a problem since overtreatment can have a negative effect on bone.

Other Vitamins and Nutrients   There appears to be little scientific evidence to support the use of unusual amounts of magnesium, zinc, or boron. Although they are important nutrients and play a role in the utilization of calcium by the body, a deficiency has not been linked to the development of osteoporosis, nor has a surplus of them been associated with preventing bone loss.[10]

OSTEOPOROSIS PREVENTION: A NECESSITY FOR ALL AGES

The natural bone loss that accompanies aging must be managed so it does not develop into the debilitating, disfiguring disease of osteoporosis. Treatment is not enough for a disease that often does not show a trace until the damage is done. Prevention must be the goal of every human being who expects to survive beyond middle age. Prevention techniques can begin at any time, but ideally the habits should form early in life. Osteoporosis prevention is dependent upon a large reserve of bone. The time to build this reserve is during childhood, adolescence, and young adulthood so that when bone loss begins after the age of 35, sufficient bone mass is present to cover the loss. Do not give up if you have reached or surpassed your middle years, because midlife bone mass can still be preserved. Preventive measures begun after osteoporosis develops may help to reduce further bone loss.

The following pages will supply information on nutrition and exercise as they apply to the prevention of osteoporosis.

Nutrition

Vitamins, minerals, and other important nutrients, in balanced proportions, are needed to keep our bodies healthy. Calcium, one of those nutrients, is essential for strong bones, but other organs such as the heart, muscles, nerves, and blood vie for the body's supply. Adequate calcium in the diet is important. The body cannot make calcium, so the diet is the sole source. Dietary intake must offset the daily losses through urine, feces (stool); and to a lesser extent sweat, skin, hair, and nails. If the level of calcium in the blood drops below normal, then calcium is taken from the bones which depletes calcium reserves. At menopause, calcium loss is increased in the urine because of increased bone resorption or loss, compounded by decreased calcium absorption in the stomach.

If calcium supply was merely dependent upon intake, maintaining that supply would be simple. Other factors affecting the supply are deficient estrogen levels, physical inactivity, excessive alcohol use, smoking, and other medical disorders.

Calcium

Calcium Intake While this section focuses primarily on the dietary requirements of calcium, keep in mind that other factors affect calcium levels. Recent national nutrition surveys have shown that the average American diet is considerably below the recommended daily allowance with regard to calcium intake. Many women and young girls, beginning as early as age 11, who diet to maintain or achieve a thin figure, consume less than half the amount of calcium recommended to grow and maintain healthy bones.[11] Males, on the other hand, seem to consume adequate amounts of calcium presumably because of their concern with physical fitness and their knowledge that diet plays a major part in the proper development and function of their bodies.

The most recent recommendations on adequate calcium intake is a result of a consensus panel convened by the National Institutes of Health (NIH) in 1994. In all age groups except for infants, the new NIH recommendations are higher than the RDA See Table 3-1

As previously noted the difference in total calcium intake for premenopausal women and estrogen-treated postmenopausal women differs because calcium is better utilized in the presence of estrogen.

Calcium is a food, not a drug, and is a "threshold" nutrient—a certain amount must be consumed in order to maintain bone mass. No one questions the need for calcium in the diet; rather, how much, in what form, and when, are the issues raised. Intake of calcium is generally safe, thanks to the mechanisms that protect most individuals against oversupply. Calcium intakes of up to 2000 mg is well tolerated, but a few individuals absorb too much calcium and may be at risk for kidney stones. For the most part, people with a history of kidney stones should avoid high intakes of calcium until they

Table 3–1
NIH Recommended Calcium Intakes

Age Group	Calcium Intake (mg/day)
Infants	
Birth–6 mo	400
6–12 mo	600
Children/Young adults	
1–10 y	800–1200
11–24 y	1200–1500
Adult women	
25–49 y	1000
50–64 y	
taking estrogen	1000
not taking estrogen	1500
65+ y	1500
Adult men	
25–64 y	1000
65+ y	1500
Pregnancy	400 mg + recommendation for specific age group

know the cause of their kidney stones. If they are in the group that absorbs too much calcium, they need to restrict their calcium intake.[11,12,13]

Calcium Sources   Adding more calcium to the diet is easy. Most experts agree that the preferred source of calcium is a nutritionally balanced diet. Food intake as a calcium source decreases the risk of consuming excessive amounts (it is difficult to consume too much calcium from usual food sources as opposed to fortified foods and pill supplements). When foods are used as a source of calcium, not only is the total content of calcium important, but also the amount that the body can absorb.

Dairy products contain a high content of readily available calcium. This means that most of the calcium that is taken in is easily absorbed and used by the body. The new food labelling process on certain specified foods shows the calcium content which in turn enables the public to select those foods rich in calcium.

For those who are on fat and calorie restricted diets, dairy food sources should not pose a problem since many sources are low in fat and calories. For example, a cup of skim milk has only 80 calories. Not only does it contain fewer calories and less fat than whole milk, it also has a greater amount of calcium. Low fat yogurt and cheese products are also high in calcium. Interestingly enough, as cheese becomes softer in consistency, the calcium content decreases. Although the primary source for calcium is found in dairy products, many other foods are also good sources of calcium. See Table 3-2.

What If I Can't Drink Milk?
Those individuals who are lactose intolerant or cannot tolerate dairy products will find they can still meet their calcium requirements. Lactose-free milk and milk substitutes are available. Lactose-containing foods can be treated with lactase drops or lactase can be taken as pills. There are even some milk products on the market that have already been treated with lactase.

Calcium, Oxalate, Phytates
Other foods such as salmon with bones, sardines, some legumes, and some green leafy vegetables are good sources of calcium, but contain less than dairy foods. Some nondairy foods that contain calcium also have oxalates and phytates which interfere with calcium absorption. Spinach, beet greens, rhubarb, and almonds are examples of foods that contain oxalates. The calcium in spinach or rhubarb is almost completely unavailable to the body. Legumes, such as pinto beans, navy beans, and peas, are high in phytates. The calcium in phytates is half as available as the calcium in milk. Phytate levels in beans can be reduced by soaking them in water for several hours, discarding the water, then cooking them in fresh water for several hours.

To derive maximum benefit from calcium-rich foods, they

Table 3-2
Keep Calcium Up And Cholesterol and Fat Down

Food Item	Serving	Calcium *mg	Cholestrol mg	Fat **g	Calories
Dairy Products					
Milk, whole	8 oz	291	33	8	150
2%	8 oz	297	18	5	121
1%	8 oz	300	10	3	102
skim	8 oz	352	5	trace	85
chocolate (2%)	8 oz	284	17	5	179
Cocoa (whole milk)	8 oz	298	33	9	218
Goat milk	8 oz	326	28	10	168
Buttermilk	8 oz	285	9	2	100
Shake, chocolate	10 oz	396	32	8	356
vanilla	11 oz	457	37	9	350
Eggnog	8 oz	330	149	19	342
Yogurt (with added milk solids)					
Plain	8 oz	274	29	7	139
Plain, low-fat	8 oz	415	14	4	145
Fruit, low-fat	8 oz	314	10	2	225
Coffee or vanilla, low-fat	8 oz	389	11	3	194
Frozen, fruit	8 oz	240	18	2	216
Frozen, chocolate	8 oz	160	17	5	220
Cheese					
Mozzarella, part skim	1 oz	207	15	5	80
Muenster	1 oz	203	27	9	105
Cheddar	1 oz	204	30	9	115
shredded	1 cup	815	119	37	455
Swiss	1 oz	272	26	8	95
American	1 oz	174	27	9	105
Ricotta, part skim	1 cup	669	76	19	340
Cottage, low-fat(2%)	1 cup	155	19	4	205
Frozen Desserts					
Ice Cream, vanilla, hard (11% fat)	1 cup	176	59	14	270
Frozen Custard	1 cup	236	153	23	375
Ice Milk, vanilla, hard (4% fat)	1 cup	176	18	6	185
Soft Serve vanilla (3% fat)	1 cup	274	13	5	225
Sherbet (2% fat)	1 cup	103	14	4	270

Table 3-2   (continued)
Keep Calcium Up And Cholesterol and Fat Down

Food Item	Serving	Calcium *mg	Cholestrol mg*	Fat **g	Calories
Fish and Shellfish					
Sardines, canned in oil, including bones	3 oz	371	85	9	175
Salmon, canned (pink), including bones	3 oz	167	34	5	120
Shrimp, canned, drained	3 oz	98	128	1	100
Oysters, fresh, raw, (13-19 med)	1 cup	226	120	4	160
Vegetables					
Broccoli, cooked,					
drained from raw	1 cup	71	0	trace	45
drained from frozen	1 cup	94	0	trace	50
Collards, cooked,					
drained from raw	1 cup	148	0	trace	25
drained from frozen	1 cup	357	0	1	60
Kale, cooked,					
drained from frozen	1 cup	179	0	1	40
Turnip Greens, cooked,					
drained from frozen	1 cup	249	0	1	50
Soybeans, cooked, drained	1 cup	131	0	10	235
Soy Products					
Tofu, piece 2½ by 2¾ by 1 in		108	0	5	85
Nuts					
Almonds, whole	1 oz	75	0	15	165
Brazil nuts, shelled	1 oz	50	0	19	185
Peanuts, roasted in oil, salted	1 oz	24	0	8	165

*mg—milligrams
**g—grams

should not be eaten at the same time as foods high in oxalates or phytates. These foods should be eaten at least an hour before or two hours following any calcium-rich foods.

Sodium and protein intake, if taken in excessive amounts, will result in calcium loss. A low sodium, low protein diet can result in a need for less calcium. Table 3-2 describes the various food sources of calcium as well as cholesterol and fat content.

What If I Don't Like Those Calcium Rich Foods?

For those whose dietary intake is inadequate, many foods and food products such as juices, fruit drinks, breads, and cereals are fortified with calcium. The labels on these products will usually indicate the amount of calcium per serving. Concerns have been raised regarding the amount of calcium available for absorption from these calcium-fortified foods, whether there is a potential for toxicity, (e.g., teenage boys who may exceed the recommended safe levels of 2000 mg/day), the possibility of an interaction with other minerals, and whether consumers are being misled into believing that intake of these foods is an adequate source for a nutritionally sound diet.[12,13]

Calcium Supplements

For those who have difficulty because of food preference, a variety of calcium supplements are available in the form of tablets. The amount of calcium needed from a supplement depends on how much calcium is obtained from food sources. For example, if a person needs 1000 mg of calcium per day, and they drink 2 cups of skim milk which gives them about 600 mg, they need only about 400 mg from a supplement. There are several different kinds of calcium preparations on the market that contain different amounts of elemental calcium, which is the actual amount of calcium in the supplement that can be used by the body. It is important to know which tablets provide the most elemental calcium and easily disintegrate in the stomach.

In the United States, calcium carbonate is the most common preparation and provides the greatest amount of elemental calcium (40 percent), and is normally the least expensive. Tablets of calcium carbonate, regardless of manufacturer, should either meet the new United States Pharmacopeia (USP) standard for disintegration or be a chewable product. The USP standards indicate that a tablet will disintegrate (break up) in the stomach.[11,12,13] Tablets that do not contain the "USP" designation or indicate their bioavailability should be avoided.[14] For the most part, the amount of calcium that can be used by the body varies among brands, but generally there are not large differences in the absorption of calcium from different calcium supplements or foods.[12,13] If in doubt, a simple test can be used to see how well a tablet will dissolve.

Test

Place a tablet in six ounces of vinegar at room temperature for about 30 minutes and stir occasionally. Tablets that dissolve in 30 minutes or less are considered satisfactory.

The body can absorb about 500 mg of calcium at any one time, whether from food or supplements. Therefore, calcium supplements are better absorbed when taken in small doses with other foods or meals several times throughout the day. Taking calcium all at once, however, is better than not taking it at all![11] Some experts even suggest consuming a calcium-rich food or supplement at bedtime to provide a calcium source during the night since the body requires calcium 24 hours a day.

Avoid taking calcium with high-fiber meals or with bulk-forming laxatives since fiber can reduce calcium absorption. Yet fiber, such as that found in fruits, vegetables, and most common cereals, seems to have no effect on calcium absorption. However, if wheat bran and calcium are taken together, absorption will be decreased.

Calcium interferes with iron absorption, so calcium and iron supplements should not be taken at the same time. See Table 3-3 for various calcium preparations.

Precautions While recommended supplements are generally safe, some precautions should be taken. For example, calcium supplements fortified with vitamin D, may lead to vitamin D toxicity if more than the recommended number of tablets are taken on a regular basis. Some preparations of calcium such as bone meal dolomite may contain lead, aluminum, arsenic, mercury, and cadmium. Previously, some

Table 3-3
Elemental Calcium Content of Some Calcium Preparation

Procuct Name	Source of Calcium (mg of avail. Calcium)	Number of tablets per day to provide approx. 1000 mg
Caltrate 600 (Lederle)	Calcium carbonate (600 mg)	1½
Caltrate 600+ 125 IU of Vitamin D (Lederle)	Calcium carbonate (600 mg)	1½
Caltrate Plus 200 IU of Vitamin D, 40 mg magnesium, 7.5 mg zinc, 1 mg copper, 1.8 mg manganese (Lederle)	Calcium carbonate (600 mg)	1½
Os-Cal 250+ 125 IU of Vitamin D (SmithKline Beecham)	Calcium carbonate (250 mg) (from oyster shell)	4
Os-Cal 500+ 125 IU of Vitamin D (SmithKline Beecham)	Calcium carbonate (500 mg) (from oyster shell)	2
Os-Cal 500 (chewable) (SmithKline Beecham)	Calcium carbonate (500 mg)	2
TUMS (SmithKline Beecham)	Calcium carbonate (200 mg)	5
TUMS E-X Tablets (SmithKline Beecham)	Calcium carbonate (300 mg)	3½
TUMS 500 (SmithKline Beecham)	Calcium carbonate (500 mg)	2
Posture (Whitehall)	Calcium carbonate (600 mg) (from Tribasic calcium phosphate)	1½
Posture-D+ 125 IU of Vitamin D (Whitehall)	Calcium carbonate (600 mg) (from Tribasic calcium phosphate)	1½
Rolaids (Warner-Lambert)	Calcium carbonate (220)	4½
Rolaids (extra-strength) (Warner-Lambert)	Calcium carbonate (400 mg)	2½
Citracal (Mission Pharmacal)	Calcium carbonate (200 mg) (from Calcium citrate)	5
Citracal+ 200 UI of Vitamin D3 (Mission Pharmacal)	Calcium carbonate (315 mg) (from Calcium citrate)	3

IU—International Units

"oyster shell" or "natural source" calcium carbonate supplements were found to have significant amounts of lead and aluminum. However, most calcium preparations are tested for heavy metal contamination and are safe.

In summary, when selecting a calcium supplement, choose one that:

- provides the most elemental calcium,
- disintegrates readily
- is manufactured by a reputable company
- is free of toxic substances

If adequate calcium cannot be obtained from the usual diet, calcium-fortified foods and calcium supplements can fill the gap to assure adequate daily calcium intake.

Table 3-3 shows both the number of milligrams and percentage of elemental calcium in the various products. The lesser the amount of calcium available in each tablet, the more tablets must be consumed to provide the required amount. If in doubt concerning the amount of elemental calcium in a product, consult a pharmacist.

Side Effects Of Calcium Supplement To prevent indigestion, constipation, and increase absorption, calcium carbonate should be taken with meals. Calcium citrate, another form of calcium, normally does not cause the gastrointestinal problems of gas, indigestion, and constipation. Try several different preparations, if necessary, to find the one that causes the least side effects. Your pharmacist can assist you. Plenty of fluids (6 to 8 glasses a day) should be consumed if you are taking a supplement.

High intake of calcium supplements may interfere with the absorption of other nutrients such as iron and zinc, and the absorption of some medications may be affected if taken at the same time as the calcium supplement. Inform your health care provider that you are currently taking calcium supplements if medication is prescribed or recommended.[12,13]

Other Factors That Interfere With Calcium Absorption

Phosphorus   Phosphorus affects the amount of calcium absorbed by the bones. Obtaining adequate amounts is usually not a problem since so many foods and beverages contain phosphorus. The problem arises when too much phosphorus is taken in, and the balance of calcium to phosphorus is affected. This results in bone breakdown, as a bone dissolving hormone is produced. Efforts should therefore be directed at decreasing the amount of phosphorus in the diet. Phosphorus

Table 3-4
Phosphorus Content of Select Foods

Food/Beverage	Serving	Phosphorus (mg)
Beverages		
Beer	12 oz	50
Coffee	6 oz	2–6
Cola (reg/diet)	12 oz	39–52
Ginger ale	12 oz	0
Grape	12 oz	0
Lemon-lime	12 oz	0
Milk (whole)	1 cup	228
Milk shake	10 oz	326–357
Orange	12 oz	4
Pepper type	12 oz	41
Root beer	12 oz	0
Tea	8 oz	2–4
Wine	3½ oz	18
Desserts (made with milk)		
Custard, frozen	1 cup	199
Ice cream (vanilla)	1 cup	134
Ice milk (vanilla)	1 cup	129
Pudding (vanilla)	½ cup	116
Fruits		
Apples	1	10
Banana	1	23
Grapefruit	½	10
Peaches	1 cup	20
Pears	1 cup	18

Table 3-4 (continued)
Phosphorus Content of Select Foods

Food/Beverage	Serving	Phosphorus (mg)
Meat and Meat Substitutes		
Beef	1 oz	65
Cheese, cheddar	1 oz	145
processed American	1 oz	211
Swiss	1 oz	171
Cottage cheese	1/4 cup	70
Cheeseburger (4 oz patty)	1 sandwich	320
Chipped Beef (dried)	2 oz	287
Egg	1	90
Fish, haddock	1 oz	68
Ham	3 oz	182
Liver	1 oz	105
Pork, lean	1 oz	70
Salami (dry type)	2 slices	28
Sandwich spread	1 tbsp	9
Peanut butter, creamy	2 Tbsp	120
Vegetables		
Beans, snap	1 cup	49
Beets	1 cup	53
Broccoli	1 cup	102
Cauliflower	1 cup	43
Peas	1 cup	144
Potato (without skin)	1	60
Starch		
Bran cereal (100%	1/2 cup	344
Bran flakes	1/2 cup	110
Bread, wheat	1 slice	65
Oatmeal, cooked	1/2 cup	90

rich foods include canned or processed meats such as hot dogs, lunch meats, bacon, ham, soft drinks, packaged pastries, cereals, breads, and instant soups. Check labels of packaged goods before buying them to determine if you are getting too much phosphorus in your diet. The RDA for females 25 years and over is 800 mg per day. Table 3-4 is an abbreviated list of the phosphorus content of foods and beverages.

Caffeine   Heavy consumers of caffeine have been found to experience greater amounts of calcium loss. Caffeine encourages the kidneys to eliminate water in the form of urine. Nutrients like calcium follow the exiting water. A moderate intake of caffeine is 400 mg per day. Beware of caffeine in other sources including various pain relievers since some contain as much as 65 mg per tablet. See Table 3-5.

High Protein Diet   A high protein diet has also been implicated in osteoporosis. Many high protein foods are also high in phosphorus which, as indicated earlier, interferes with calcium utilization. High levels of both protein and sodium in the diet are thought to increase calcium excretion or loss. Excessive amounts of these substances should be avoided un-

Table 3-5
Caffeine Content of Select Beverage, Foods, and Medications

Food/Beverage/Medicine	Serving	Caffeine (mg)
Coffee		
drip-brewed	5-oz cup	30–180
instant	5-oz cup	50–110
decaffeinated	5-oz cup	2–5
Tea		
black, green	5-oz cup	2–110 (average: 30–60)
decaffeinated	5-oz cup	1
Soft Drinks	12-oz	35–50
Cocoa	5-oz	2–20
Chocolate		
Syrup	1 oz	4
Cake	$1/16$ piece	15
Ice Cream	$1/2$ cup	5
pudding	$1/2$ cup	4–8
Milk Chocolate	1-oz piece	1–15
Aspirin (Bayer, select)	1 caplet	65
Aspirin Free Excedrin	1 caplet	65
Excedrin	1 caplet	65
Vanquish	1 caplet	65
Vivarin	1 caplet	200
No Doz	1 caplet	200

til more studies are conducted to determine safe intake levels.[11] Total sodium intake should not exceed 2400 mg daily. The Food Guide Pyramid in Chapter 6 will assist you in the selection of the appropriate amounts and kinds of protein sources.

Tobacco   Tobacco smoke interferes with the liver's ability to use estrogen. If estrogen is needed for proper calcium utilization and cigarettes interfere with this process, the higher incidence of osteoporosis in smokers is plausible.

Alcohol   Decreased calcium absorption has also been found in heavy drinkers, although the precise level at which alcohol intake increases the risk of osteoporosis is not well established. Heavy drinkers usually have poor dietary habits so their calcium intake is probably poor as well. Nevertheless, a high consumption of alcohol on a regular basis is detrimental not only to bone health but to health in general. For women, "moderate drinking" is no more than one drink per day, according to the U.S. Dietary guidelines for Americans and includes:

- 12 ounces of regular beer
- 5 ounces of wine
- $1^{1}/_{2}$ ounces of hard liquor (80 proof)

Why The Controversy In The Use Of Calcium?

Increasing calcium intake alone cannot solve the osteoporosis problem, because osteoporosis is not a simple condition. Many factors are responsible and these multiple factors make it difficult to evaluate the studies that have been conducted thus far. The inconsistencies can be explained by the following:

- Bone is a complex structure. A number of factors in addition to calcium are responsible for bone health. Therefore, using calcium as a measurement of bone health may be ineffective if there are other causative factors aside from calcium.

- Calcium deficiency can be the result of inadequate calcium intake or poor absorption and utilization, thus increasing intake alone may not be sufficient. How the body absorbs and gets rid of calcium excess differs among individuals. Some individuals may have problems absorbing calcium and therefore will need greater amounts.

- The ability to absorb calcium effectively declines with age.

- The length of time since menopause and the effect of estrogen deficiency on bone loss are influences on study results. Menopausal age and calcium intake status are influential factors in bone density and bone loss studies, because bone loss is believed to be greatest during the first five to ten years following menopause. Increased calcium has the greatest impact on bone density for approximately six years postmenopause and also in those individuals whose calcium intake is low.

- The availability of vitamin D, which is important in the absorption of calcium, decreases as one ages.

- Measuring bone mass and calcium intake is difficult. Current bone mass is the result of past, not current calcium intake; and current calcium intake does not necessarily reflect past calcium intake.

- Studies are time consuming. A minimum of two years is required to adequately determine whether calcium intake has had an effect on bone density.

At this point you should have some insight into some of the discrepancies that you may see or hear with regard to the use of calcium. Nevertheless, a consensus seems to exist that low calcium intakes are associated with low bone mass, rapid bone loss, and high fracture rates. And an adequate intake of calcium is important in the bone formation years—childhood and young adulthood.

Vitamin D, Magnesium, And Vitamin C

Vitamin D   A great deal of attention has been paid to the roles of vitamin D and magnesium and their relationship to calcium. Many calcium supplements are available with vitamin D. Vitamin D plays a major role in calcium absorption and its incorporation into bone. The body manufactures this vitamin as a result of exposure to sunlight. For most people, an unrestricted diet and some exposure to sunlight provide adequate amounts of vitamin D. Foods such as salmon, mackerel, halibut, eggs, butter, liver, and vitamin D enriched milk will also provide sufficient quantities.

Too much vitamin D is harmful, so supplements in excess of 400 international units (IU), the U.S. RDA, should never be taken without the advice of a health professional. Doses greater than 800 IU/day favor bone loss and can contribute to heart or muscle problems.

Individuals who are at risk for vitamin D deficiency are the very old, those with chronic disease, and those who are home-bound with little or no sun exposure. Usually, a multi-vitamin with 400 IU of vitamin D daily is adequate for both the home-bound and those who live in climates with minimal sun exposure.

Magnesium   Magnesium is a mineral which has been found to be instrumental in converting vitamin D to its usable form and maintaining calcium in the bloodstream. Magnesium is abundant in green leafy vegetables, nuts, and whole-grain cereals, legumes, and seafoods. Little evidence of magnesium deficiency in the general population exists, thus there is no need for additional intake except in severe, prolonged vomiting, cirrhosis of the liver, chronic alcoholism, and severe malabsorption diseases such as ulcerative colitis and Crohn's disease.

Vitamin C   Vitamin C is also essential in proper bone formation. As one ages, the need for vitamin C increases to aid in bone and supportive tissue reconstruction. With age, less acid is produced in the stomach, diminishing adequate calcium absorption. Vitamin C creates a weak acid environment which helps the absorption of calcium. A well balanced diet will provide adequate amounts (60 mg per day is the RDA).

An unstable material, vitamin C is easily destroyed by

exposure to air, so eating foods when they are as fresh as possible is the best way to get the most vitamin C. Vitamin loss from fresh fruits and vegetables is reduced when these foods are stored in the refrigerator and vegetables steamed. See Table 3-6.

Exercise

According to gynecologist, Dr. Mona Shangold, Director of the Sports Gynecology and Women's Life Cycle Center at Hahnemann University, "Although many women over age 50 believe exercise is dangerous for them, it is actually dangerous for them not to exercise." A modest program of weight-bearing and strength building exercise is recommended for people of all ages, including middle-aged and older women, and young women who are working toward reaching a high "peak bone mass" in their mid-thirties. No one is ever too old to start some kind of exercise program, and even those affect-

Table 3-6
Vitamin C Content of Select Foods

Food	Serving	mg ascorbic acid
Beef liver	3 oz	23
Broccoli	½ cup	50
Cabbage, cooked	½ cup	36
Cantaloupe	½ cup	90
Cauliflower	½ cup	30
Grapefruit		
fresh	1	41
juice	½ cup	42
Orange		
fresh	1	70
juice	½ cup	49
Potato, boiled	1	18
Spinach, cooked	1 cup	29
Strawberries, whole, fresh	½ cup	42
Tomato		
raw	1	22
juice	1 cup	39
Turnip greens	½ cup	20

ed with osteoporosis will benefit from exercise. Lack of activity seems to do more harm than good both physically and mentally. Even individuals with osteoporosis are encouraged to remain as physically active as possible with certain restrictions. According to most experts, one of the worst things an individual with osteoporosis can do is to give in and "take to one's bed or chair."

Exercise Prevention   Exercise is important in an osteoporosis prevention and treatment program. Not only does it improve bone health, but it also improves muscle strength, coordination, balance, and overall physical health.[15] It is now well established that mechanical forces and physical activity influence bone mass. Physical inactivity, such as prolonged bedrest, even in normal healthy people causes bone loss. In fact, complete bedrest can cause loss of bone tissue by as much as 4% per month. Living in a weightless environment, such as in space flights, also causes bone loss. Conversely, athletes, who exercise more often and more consistently than the average person, usually have above-average bone mass.[16] Higher bone density has been found in experienced runners than in sedentary individuals. Not only is bone density higher in physically active people, increased activity is also associated with lower rates of age-related bone loss. Studies on older athletic women found their bone density to be similar to those of younger athletes. "Athletic" adult women were those who exercised at least three times per week, 8 or more months of the year for a minimum of 3 years.[17]

What Are The Forces At Work?   The positive effect of weight bearing on bone density has long been recognized. New studies indicate that non-weight bearing, muscle-stretching exercises such as swimming and biking also encourage bone density. Studies conducted on women who supplemented aerobic exercise with one hour of weight training had higher spine densities when compared to those who engaged only in aerobic exercise. Furthermore, swimming, which is a nonweight-bearing activity, has been known to contribute to increased bone density through the high intensity muscular activity. Likewise, improved bone mass in the spine has been found with use of a stationary cycle. Although these alternatives deserve further study, their merit lies with the fact that they apparently contribute to a favorable effect, even though intensity and duration are yet to be decided.

More Questions

Bone Formation Although the relationship of physical activity to bone vitality is not completely understood, one plausible explanation is that mechanical stress alters the electrical charge on bone surfaces which, in turn, activates bone forming cells. This stress appears to have a localized effect and suggests that an exercise program should involve activities that add mechanical stress to the areas where osteoporotic fractures occur most frequently, such as the spine, hip, and wrist.

- A study conducted on postmenopausal women who participated in a program of arm exercises showed bone density of the wrist increased in these women as opposed to nonexercising women who lost bone density.
- Other studies have shown that engaging in regular weight-bearing exercise increases hip bone density.
- Furthermore, studies that have used varied exercise programs which included aerobics, calisthenics, and stair climbing, have found increases in bone density of the spine.

Thus, activities such as jogging, brisk walking, stair climbing, or dancing have an effect on both hip and spinal bone density. What all of this tells us is that bone density can be increased at any site if adequate stress is provided to that bone (or to the muscles attached to it).

Other Benefits

A physically fit body provides additional rewards. Exercise programs that benefit bone can also strengthen muscles and improve balance and coordination which reduces the chances of falling and fracturing a bone.

Decreased Bone Loss

Finally, although estrogen deficiency appears to be the most important cause of bone loss in the postmenopausal woman, inactivity is detrimental as well. What follows are several different types of activities and ways to get yourself started on the road to bone health.

Bone Saving Fitness Plan

Prior to beginning an exercise program, there are some general steps to take.

See A Health Care Provider   Before beginning any exercise program, schedule a comprehensive medical examination with your health care provider, especially if heart, joint, or other problems exist. Prolonged inactivity also requires an examination before beginning an exercise program.

Be Prepared   No matter what exercise you choose, be sure to select the proper equipment and footwear.

Build Gradually   Begin your exercise routine slowly and build gradually so that your heart, lungs, and muscles can adapt to the new demands you are placing on them.

Listen To Your Body   Since it takes time for muscles to become conditioned, a little stiffness or soreness can be expected and is normal. Pain is not normal. Do not overexert yourself.

Choose A Convenient Place To Exercise   It may be a health club or an exercise program at home. Whatever works best for you, videotapes or exercise equipment such as cycles, steppers, rowing machines, or treadmills will achieve the same effect as a health club or outside activities. Add music or television to your indoor home program to break up the monotony and keep yourself motivated!

Schedule Your Time Plan to exercise thirty minutes, three to four times a week. Pick one or several sports such as walking, jogging, weight training, stair climbing or "steppers," soccer, lacrosse, field hockey, tennis, racquet ball, squash, basketball, volleyball, dancing, swimming, bicycling, or skiing. Do not be discouraged thinking these activities are only for the "young." Desire, not age, drives physical activity. Common sense warns not to start out with field hockey, lacrosse or 10 mile run when the most exercise you've had in the past 15 years has been walking from your car to a destination 200 feet away. Start out slowly and progress at your own speed.

Design A Fitness Game Plan Select activities you find enjoyable.

Plan A Daily Routine Exercise should be so much a part of your life that you feel guilty if forced to miss the activity. Vary your routine to add interest.

Participate In Low Impact Activates For individuals with established osteoporosis, activities such as walking are beneficial. Care and planning must come first to avoid possible falls.

No magic formula for duration, frequency, and intensity of activities has been discovered. The benefits of 30 to 60 minute workout sessions have been verified, but little information exists on the benefits of shorter segments. If short periods are all you can handle, then spend the time you can. Once that routine is set, you may just find additional time.

Variety Is The "Spice Of Life"

A program that alternates activities not only avoids boredom, but also "works" various parts of the body. For example, walking is good for the legs, heart, and lungs, but results in decreased muscle tone and strength in the trunk and upper body. Therefore "Wall Pushups", "Triceps and Biceps Curls", "Shoulder Presses", and "Kickbacks", as shown in Figure 3-9 are one group of options to build upper body strength. One-, two- and three-pound weights are desirable for women who want to tone, rather than build muscle mass.

Of course the activity that is chosen depends upon an individual's likes, dislikes, and availability of space and equipment. If tennis, racquet ball, or jogging are out of the question for you, then perhaps brisk walking, dancing, aerobics and/or weight lifting is more appealing. Indoor options should also be considered for those times of the year when inclement weather prevents outside activities.

It has been found that gains in bone mass are lost when physical activity is discontinued, thus it is important to develop an exercise program that is workable and fits into your usual schedule.

Ideally, prevention of osteoporosis should start early with regular exercise in young women to maintain "peak bone mass" throughout the mature adult years.

Keep the following guidelines in mind as you perform the following weight-lifting exercises in the "Bone-Saving Fitness Plan" in Figure 3-9.

- Do the routine three days a week; it shouldn't take more than 15 to 20 minutes

- Take a day off in between workouts because muscles need to rest.

- You may combine your weight lifting with other exercise programs such as walking, jogging etc.

- Perform each exercise slowly and deliberately; do not let the weight drop as you lower it.

- Breathe out through your mouth as you lift, and in as you lower, keeping your stomach muscles pulled in.

- For each exercise, start with one set of eight repetitions, using a weight that allows you to do this many repetitions without getting so fatigued that you lose your form. As soon as eight repetitions of any exercise become easy, add another set. Once that becomes easy, increase your weight, going back to one set of eight repetitions. Continue this pattern until you feel you may need heavier weights or continue at a level that works best for you. Consistency is key!

Wall Push-Ups (Upper body/wrists)

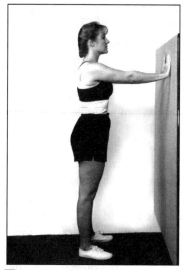 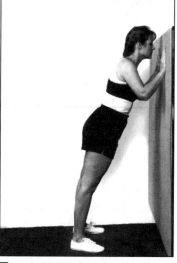

A Stand an arm's length from wall, feet shoulder width apart. Place hands on wall shoulder distance apart, fingers pointing up.

B Bend elbows, keeping torso straight and heels on floor, until forehead almost touches wall. Straighten arms and push against wall to return to starting position.

Shoulder Press (Deltoids)

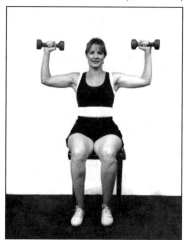 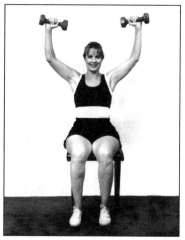

A Sit on stool, legs relaxed, stomach taut. Holding a weight in each hand, palms facing forward, raise arms to shoulder level and bend elbows 90 degrees.

B Lift weights straight overhead; don't lock elbows. Slowly lower weights to starting position.

Kick Back (Triceps)

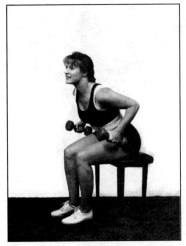 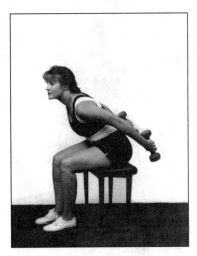

A Lean forward slightly on stool, a weight in each hand. With arm bent, lift elbows straight behind you, keeping shoulders relaxed.

B Straighten arms, keeping upper arms still and close to body. Slowly bend elbows to starting position.

Chest Squeeze

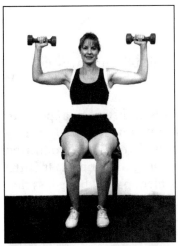 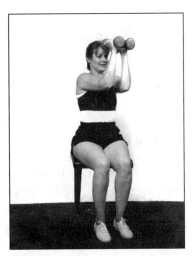

A Hold a weight in each hand, palms facing forward; raise arms to shoulder level and bend elbows 90 degrees.

B Without changing position of arms, bring weights and elbows together in front of body, squeezing chest as you do so.

Biceps Curls

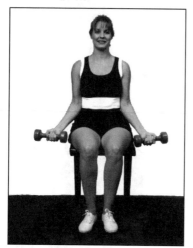 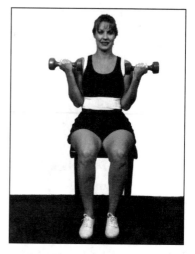

A Holding a weight in each hand, sit with arms straight, palms facing forward, elbows next to waist.

B Bend elbows, keeping upper arms steady, until weights almost touch shoulders. Slowly lower weights, resisting gravity, to starting position.

Figure 3-9

Source: "The Bone-Saving Fitness Plan". This article was first published in *Season's* magazine which appeared in Volume 3 Issue 5. Adapted with permission.

BONE HEALTH SUMMARY

Evidence exists that suggests bone health improves in post-menopausal women who increase their calcium intake.[18] How helpful increased calcium intake alone is for protecting bone density is somewhat controversial. Estrogen appears to be the dominant factor since calcium is not utilized well by the bones in its absence. This decrease in estrogen production greatly accelerates the loss of bone in most women. It is the five to ten year period of rapid postmenopausal bone loss that probably accounts for the high proportion of women with osteoporosis. There does appear to be some evidence that increased calcium intake, especially for the first five years after menopause, or after the acute menopausal phase, helps to maintain bone. Yet, it is also known, even megadoses of calcium cannot compare with estrogen therapy in successfully preventing bone loss.[19,20] Thus, most of the information that is available seems to indicate that, replacement with calcium alone is insufficient to prevent bone loss in most postmenopausal women, and calcium supplementation alone is not an alternative to estrogen therapy for prevention of osteoporosis.

However, for those who cannot take estrogen to prevent osteoporosis, a balanced diet rich in calcium is needed throughout one's lifetime, since, normally, it can do no harm, and any positive effect is better than nothing at all. Furthermore, a decreased intake of caffeine, phosphorus and protein combined with a weight-bearing exercise program are additional steps to promote bone health. Discretion with alcohol use, smoking cessation, and monitoring drugs which may interfere with calcium absorption or loss will further enhance a bone conservation program. Many dietary and exercise suggestions made throughout this book will benefit any woman who chooses not to, or is unable to take hormone therapy.

Bone Health Tips For Women

- hormone replacement therapy
- calcitonin to slow bone breakdown
- calcium
  - 1000 mg daily for postmenopausal women on HRT
  - 1500 mg daily for postmenopausal women not on HRT
- etidronate/alendronate for treatment of osteoporosis
- regular weight-bearing exercise which causes muscles to work against gravity (walking, stair climbing, "steppers," jogging, tennis, aerobics, dancing)
  - walk short distances instead of driving
  - use steps instead of an elevator when possible
  - do house and yard work
- weight-lifting activities such as carrying your own luggage and groceries when possible

- other forms of exercise such as cycling, rowing, and swimming may benefit your bones and also have cardiovascular benefits

- exercise also plays a role in weight control and makes it easier to maintain an adequate intake of calcium and other nutrients

- the more you sit, the more you need exercise

- avoid smoking and use moderation with alcoholic beverages [20,21,22]

- make your environment safe to avoid falls

DO NOT FORGET TEENS AND MEN

During the teenage years, hormones (estrogen in girls and testosterone in boys) help bones grow in size and strength. Much more bone is deposited than withdrawn until around 25 to 35. Prior to this time is when bones reach their maximum strength and density.

A large bank account of bone tissue is needed to draw from when one gets older. As women age their production of estrogen decreases, and they lose a great deal of bone tissue. Although men do not stop producing testosterone, they do experience bone loss, but at a far slower rate than women. Therefore, the teen years are the best time to build up the "bank account" so there will be plenty of bone to "withdraw" from when the time comes.[22,23]

Bone Health Tips For Teens
- The best way to prevent osteoporosis when you get older is to build strong bones NOW with a balanced diet rich in calcium and an active life style.

- Dieting can keep you from getting calcium and other nutrients.

  - Starving yourself to lose weight (a disorder called anorexia nervosa), or use of laxatives and measures which induce vomiting (a disorder called bulimia), can be very serious and lead to osteoporosis and broken bones.

- Calcium intake can be increased without causing weight gain.

- To increase your calcium intake, try the following:

  - have cheese on your burgers, or add cheese to salads

  - have low-fat yogurt, frozen yogurt, or ice milk for dessert

  - snack on broccoli with dip

  - drink milk or milk shakes instead of soft drinks

  - use low-fat cheeses and yogurt, and skim milk whenever possible

- Don't be a couch potato, bones need exercise to grow and stay healthy just as muscles do.

- The following weight-bearing exercises help to build strong bones:

  - walking—walk to school or other places rather than driving or riding

  - take the stairs rather than the elevator

  - try jogging, weight lifting, or play tennis, soccer, volleyball, or basketball

  - take dance classes

  - housework and yard work—physical work is great for building bones, and makes you very popular at home!

- Physical activity of any kind is good for your bones and exercise burns calories, all of which allows you to keep your weight under control and stay healthy at the same time.

- Avoid alcohol and smoking since both of these can be harmful to your bones by slowing bone growth and damaging bone tissue.[23,24]

Bone Health For Men Of All Ages

Although women lose bone mass rapidly in the years following menopause, by age 65 or 70 men lose bone at almost the same rate as women and calcium absorption decreases in both sexes. Although men do not experience menopause, the male hormone testosterone plays an important role in bone health and a decrease can cause reduced bone mass which can lead to fractures. Risk factors linked to osteoporosis in men include:

- A decrease in the male hormone testosterone ether through the aging process or in younger men, as a result of certain medical conditions.

- Glucocorticoid medications which are used in the treatment of asthma, arthritis and Crohn's disease interfere with normal bone and calcium metabolism.

- Excessive use of alcohol reduces levels of testosterone and seems to play a role in weakening bones even in younger men; studies have also found a higher intake of alcohol and cigarette use in men with osteoporosis.

Bone Health Tips For Men
- Balanced diet rich in calcium throughout lifetime; or use of calcium fortified foods or supplements; 1000 mg per day for those under 65, and 1500 mg for those over 65

- Regular weight-bearing exercise which cause muscles to work against gravity (walking, tennis, dancing)
  - walk when you can rather than driving
  - do housework and yard work
  - use stairs whenever possible rather than an elevator

- Other forms of exercise such as cycling, rowing, and swimming may benefit your bones and also have cardiovascular benefits

- the more you sit, the more you need to exercise!

- exercise also plays a role in weight control and makes it easier to maintain an adequate intake of calcium and other nutrients

- make the environment safe to avoid falls.[24,25]

OSTEOPOROSIS AND THE FEMALE ATHLETE

Much has been said about the advantages of exercise. Certainly young women are encouraged to participate in competitive sports, but excessive exercise and intense physical training may lead to serious health consequences. A relationship has been found between excessive exercise and cessation or lack of menstruation. Competitive physical activities such as running, ballet dancing, and gymnastics have demonstrated such a relationship when young women exercise to the point that they stop menstruating or their menstrual periods become irregular. Any beneficial effect of exercise is overcome, and significant bone loss begins. It seems that infrequent and irregular or absent periods are more prevalent among athletes (10 to 20%) than among the general population (5%).[26] A good example of this is seen in studies of runners with normal menstrual periods as compared with those who stopped menstruation. Runners without periods usually ran further and more frequently, had lower bone density, and lower estrogen and progesterone levels than runners with normal menstrual periods. Furthermore, bone density in these same individuals was similar to that of 50 year old women. Stress fractures, which occur mostly in the legs, have also been found in athletes with menstrual irregularities and low bone density.

Although the association between exercise-associated amenorrhea (absence of menstrual periods) and decreased bone mass is not precisely clear, several factors such as decreased estrogen levels and inadequate calorie and calcium intake may play a role. Individuals who start endurance training at an early age are more susceptible to amenorrhea; therefore, their bones never reach the same density and strength as those athletes who continue to menstruate. Since peak bone density is related to circulating estrogen levels, girls with diminished estrogen levels due to excess exercise will reach their peak bone mass years with low bone density and will be more susceptible to osteoporosis. This is yet another reason why osteoporosis is often considered a pediatric disease.[26,27]

Decreasing the intensity and frequency of any of these excessive exercise activities usually results in a return of normal menstrual periods and subsequent increase in bone mass. What is still not known is whether this return to "normalcy" occurs when individuals have been without menstrual periods for several years.

The area of osteoporosis research in young females is comparatively new. The best advice for women who participate in any kind of athletic activity, whether it be ballet, gymnastics, running, or other types of endurance training is not to train to the extent that menstrual function either becomes irregular or menstrual periods stop.

OSTEOPOROSIS AND ANOREXIA NERVOSA

Anorexia nervosa is an eating disorder that is relatively common in young women, but less so in young men. It is characterized by severe weight loss in the absence of any obvious physical cause. The severe weight loss is caused by self-imposed starvation. One of the effects of this weight loss is amenorrhea. Of major importance is that this disorder may occur not only in adult women, but also in adolescent and preadolescent girls who are in the process of developing maximal bone mass. Many studies have shown that osteoporosis develops in young women with anorexia nervosa. The bone loss these individuals sustain is far worse than that of the athlete. In addition to estrogen deficiency, there are a number of other nutritional and hormonal influences that affect bone mass. Unfortunately, even though the prevalence of anorexia nervosa and eating disorders is on the increase, few studies exist that explain what happens to bone mass in women who recover from these disorders, and how bone mass can be preserved or increased. Studies conducted thus far suggest that a significant number of young women with a history of this eating disorder may have a permanent reduction in their bone mass which will continue to put them at risk for osteoporosis throughout the remainder of their life.[28]

IT IS NEVER TOO EARLY OR TOO LATE TO START

Preventative methods and good health habits can begin at

anytime during the life cycle. Solid nutrition and adequate exercise can always improve emotional outlook and energy levels. Osteoporosis can be combatted with an improved lifestyle. Yet the ultimate goal for prevention is to start during the early years to foster good bone formation. Parents have long been aware of the effects of good nutrition, but unfortunately teenagers usually take control of their own dietary regime with inadequate diets as the result. Cognizant of this fact, the National Institutes of Health has recommended a higher calcium intake for children and young adults in order to protect against future bone loss. Education will not only protect adults from the debilitating effects of osteoporosis, but will also aid adults in protecting and teaching future generations.

Women And Cardiovascular (Heart) Disease

The notion that cardiovascular disease afflicts only men is unfounded and completely incorrect. Heart disease stands as the number one killer of men and women. Symptoms in women appear five to ten years later than for men, but the fact that they can appear is important to health planning. Prior to menopause, the death and disability rates related to cardiovascular disease in women are relatively low; after menopause the rates increase sharply. Check the numbers for women alone![1,2]

- One in ten American women 45-64 years of age has some form of heart disease.
- One in five women over age 65 has some form of heart disease.
- The death rate from cardiovascular disease for women ages 55 to 59 is over 50 times the rate of women 30 to 34 years of age.
- Cardiovascular disease kills more women than all forms of cancer combined.
- In the United States, an estimated 625,000 women have heart attacks annually.

The cardiovascular system is made up of the heart, the blood vessels (arteries, veins, capillaries), and the blood. Statistics support how easily this system's balance can be upset.[1]

- Every year, since 1900, cardiovascular disease has been the number one killer in the United States (the influenza epidemic of 1918 is the only exception).

- The death rate for cardiovascular disease still ranks ahead of cancer deaths, accidental deaths, and deaths caused by HIV (AIDS).

WHAT IS HEART DISEASE?

Cardiovascular disease or heart disease are general terms used to describe serious disorders of the heart and blood vessels. The diseases of the cardiovascular system are often difficult to manage. Therefore, prevention is the best defense in combating these diseases. Research has helped. The death rate from cardiovascular disease in 1950 was 424 per 100,000 as opposed to 186 per 100,000 in 1991. Unfortunately, most cardiovascular research has studied the relationship of men to the disease and not women. New efforts are being made to open research doors to the study of women. In the meantime, women should educate themselves about cardiovascular disease.

Coronary heart disease is a disease of the blood vessels of the heart and causes heart attacks.When a heart attack occurs, oxygen and nutrients cannot get to the heart because of a blockage in an artery. Strokes occur when either bleeding occurs in the brain or when enough blood cannot get to the brain. Other kinds of cardiovascular disease are high blood pressure (hypertension), angina (chest pain), and rheumatic heart disease.

Heart Attack

A heart attack in medical terms is referred to as a "myocardial infarction." When women have a sudden or acute heart attack, the outlook is usually more serious than for men. In fact, the first heart attack for women is more often fatal; but if women do survive, they tend to respond more poorly to treatment than men.

First Attack   The first heart attack for women is more serious than the first attack for men because women usually experience heart attacks at an older age than men. Approximately 20% of women die within an hour after their heart attack starts—usually before they have received medical help. Those who experience this first attack at an older age are twice as likely as men to have a poor recovery.

Time Age works against women, but so does time. Minutes count when a person has a medical emergency like a heart attack. When experiencing signs and symptoms of a heart attack, women are known to delay medical treatment much longer than men do. In an ideal situation, treatment would be started within an hour after symptoms begin; however, most people delay an average of four hours before seeking medical care.Women wait even longer if they live that long!

Warning Signs Of A Heart Attack When the natural balance of the cardiovascular system is upset, the body attempts to alert the person before disaster strikes. The body sends out any number of signs warning of a heart attack. These signals often occur with physical activity, but may occur at rest. They also may come and go. Everyone should be familiar with the warning signs of a heart attack, but individuals with any risk factors should be especially alert. Risk factors include

- a family history where a family member experiences heart disease before the age of 55
- age; the older you are the greater your risk, although women in their 50s may also have heart attacks
- race; the African-American race has a higher risk for both heart disease and stroke than White women
- smoking
- high blood pressure
- high cholesterol and triglycerides
- overweight
- physical inactivity
- diabetes
- an easily stressed personality

Having any of the risk factors does not mean that you have or will develop cardiovascular disease, but the likelihood is increased. If you have any two risk factors and experience any of the following signals for longer than 10 minutes—think "heart attack":

- generalized weakness (weakness all over)
- shortness of breath
- tightness, pressure pain, or burning in the chest
- pain or discomfort in the shoulder, neck, jaw, or either arm
- sweating in combination with any of these
- nausea

Remember, women do not always have the same intensity or kinds of symptoms that men do, so if you have any of the above symptoms, **SEEK MEDICAL HELP IMMEDIATELY.** Do not hesitate since the risk of dying from a heart attack is greatest in the first few hours.

Stroke
A heart attack is not the only result of cardiovascular disease. A stroke may also occur. Nearly 1.6 million women have had a stroke while 90,000 women die each year of this condition.[3]

Who Gets Cardiovascular Disease?
In childhood, cardiovascular disease is rare and if present is usually due to congenital heart disease (a defect present at birth); and the occurrence in young boys and girls is almost equal. As early as 20 to 30 years of age, the male to female risk increases and continues to be twice as high in men until about 40 to 50 years of age. At about 40 to 50 years of age the risk increase is greater in women, and reaches almost equal occurrence in males and females at about 70 to 90 years of age.

Age Groups Some groups of women are more likely to develop cardiovascular disease. For example, Black women from ages 35 to 74 have a death rate from heart attack that is about two times that of White women, and their death rate from stroke is much higher. Age is a definite factor since older women are more likely to suffer from high blood pressure, high blood cholesterol levels, diabetes, overweight, and physical inactivity than younger women.

Menopausal Women Medical evidence links estrogen to cardiovascular disease. After menopause, women seem to develop cardiovascular diseases because their bodies produce less estrogen. Even women who have an early menopause, either naturally or surgically as a result of a hysterectomy, are twice as likely to develop coronary heart disease as women of the same age who have not begun menopause.

Count The Risk Factors While any one risk factor will raise your chances of developing heart-related problems, the more risk factors you have, the more concerned you should be about prevention. For example, if you smoke cigarettes and have high blood pressure, your chance of developing coronary heart disease increases dramatically. Having all three major risk factors—smoking, high blood pressure, and high blood cholesterol—can boost your risk to eight times that of women who have no risk factors. The good news about these risk factors is that, for the most part, they can be changed by taking an active role in your own heart health.[4]

MAJOR RISK FACTORS

The risk factors discussed in detail in this section are high blood cholesterol, high blood pressure, and smoking. All of these factors can be managed with proper knowledge and action.

High Blood Cholesterol

Cholesterol is a fat-like substance known as a lipid. The food we eat and the body itself maintains the human system's supply of cholesterol. The liver produces cholesterol daily. A certain level of cholesterol is necessary for the health of the nervous system and brain, and the production of certain hormones. A soft, waxy, fat-like substance, cholesterol, can be found only in foods that come from animals—that is, all meats and dairy products. Organ meats, such as liver, brain, and kidney, are concentrated sources of cholesterol. Egg yolks also contain a significant amount of cholesterol. Plant foods such as grains, vegetables, fruits, and nuts contain no cholesterol. Knowing which foods contain cholesterol is beneficial in planning your daily meals. Table 3-2 lists the fat, cholesterol, calcium, and calorie content of some popular foods.

Too Much Cholesterol Although the body needs cholesterol to function normally, too much of certain types of cholesterol can lead to cardiovascular disease. Excess cholesterol and other fatty materials deposit themselves on the walls of blood vessels. As these deposits grow, the blood vessels become narrower and narrower, allowing less blood to pass. If the blood vessels affected are arteries which supply oxygen and nutrients to the body, then the tissues supplied by these arteries suffer. If the arteries affected supply the heart, then the heart is weakened and heart disease results.

Cholesterol Measurements Persons with high blood cholesterol can be identified with a simple blood test that measures total blood cholesterol. Cholesterol levels are measured in milligrams of cholesterol per deciliter of blood or mg/dL. For all adults, a desirable level of total blood cholesterol is less than 200 mg/dL. Young women tend to have lower cholesterol levels than young men. Blood cholesterol levels among women begin to rise higher than men's between the ages of 45 and 55. After age 55, the gap between men and women's cholesterol level widens even more so.

The higher the blood cholesterol level, the higher the risk for heart disease. So much so that women between ages 45 and 74 who have a cholesterol level over 240 mg/dL are more than twice as likely to develop coronary heart disease as women with levels below 200 mg/dL.[4] However, even "borderline" levels between 200 and 239 increase one's risk of coronary heart disease. See Table 4-1.

HDL Versus LDL Merely knowing a total blood cholesterol level is not enough. Low-density lipoproteins (LDL) and high-density lipoproteins (HDL) affect cholesterol levels. If total blood cholesterol levels are high or even borderline and other heart disease risk factors such as smoking and high blood pressure exist, a "cholesterol profile" will usually be performed which measures both LDL and HDL levels.

Test Results Understanding the relationship of LDL to HDL can be confusing, so take some time reviewing these ideas. An LDL level below 130 mg/dL is desirable, 130 to 159 mg/dL levels are "borderline-high," and 160 mg/dL or above indicates a high risk for developing coronary heart disease. The lower the HDL number, the higher the risk for coronary heart disease. An HDL level below 35 mg/dL is considered too low; whereas, if the level is 60 or above, there is a lower risk of developing heart disease.

The Functions Of HDL And LDL LDLs carry excess cholesterol which leads to a buildup of harmful deposits in the arteries. This function has earned LDLs the title of "bad" cholesterol. The HDLs are considered "good" cholesterol because, far from being killers, they may actually play an important role in preventing heart disease. HDL helps remove cholesterol from the blood, preventing it from piling up in the arteries. HDL seems to act like a biological vacuum cleaner, sucking up excess cholesterol in the bloodstream. Cholesterol is transported away from the arteries to the liver, where it is recycled or eliminated.

Menopause And Bad Cholesterol Until about age 55 (until the postmenopause), LDL cholesterol levels are lower in women than in men. After age 55, the relationship is reversed. From then onward, women have higher HDL levels than do men of the same age, and the rates of heart disease increase tenfold for women 55 years or older as compared with women 35 to 54 years of age.[5,6]

Three known causes of elevated levels of LDL are

- family history
- a diet high in cholesterol and saturated fats
- diseases such as liver disease, diabetes, kidney disease, and an underactive thyroid

Causes of low HDL levels may include

- high total blood cholesterol or triglycerides
- obesity/overweight
- lack of exercise
- smoking

Table 4-1
Blood Cholesterol Levels

	Desirable	Borderline-High	High
Total	under 200 mg	200-239 mg	240 mg and above
LDL	under 130 mg	130-159 mg	160 mg and above
HDL	over 35 mg is ideal		

A ratio between total cholesterol and good cholesterol can be calculated by dividing the total cholesterol by the good cholesterol. If the ratio is under 4.0, your risk is not high.

EXAMPLE: (total)   (HDL)   (ratio)
240 ÷ 50 = 4.8

Fat Finding
Cholesterol levels are affected not only by the body's production of cholesterol, but also by the total fat dietary intake. This notion introduces several new terms and ideas that will

be discussed in this section. The terms are saturated fat, unsat-urated fat, polyunsaturated, monounsaturated, and triglyc-erides.

Saturated Versus Unsaturated Fats   The sources of saturated and unsaturated fats in our diet differ greatly. Understanding their sources can help protect against high cholesterol levels since intake of saturated fat tends to raise blood cholesterol levels while unsaturated fats may help to lower blood choles-terol levels.

Saturated Fats   Saturated fats are fats that become solid at room temperature. They boost your blood cholesterol level more than anything else in your diet, and are usually found in animal products such as meats, eggs, whole milk, hard cheeses, and butter. Although intake of fat from animal sources has decreased over the past 40 years, the greatest amount of fat in the average American diet still comes from meat, fish, and poultry. Much attention has focused on saturated versus unsat-urated fats and what causes the most harm.

Unsaturated Fats   Unsaturated fats do not raise blood cho-lesterol and occur chiefly in vegetable sources such as saf-flower, corn, cottonseed, soybean, and sunflowers. They are usually in a soft or liquid form. Oils contain large amounts of unsaturated fats, with the exception of coconut, palm, and palm-kernel oils, which are highly saturated. Attention must be paid when using unsaturated fat products like margarine and shortening because unsaturated oils are sometimes put through a process which makes them become more saturated. Unsaturated fats may be listed on labels as polyunsaturated or monounsaturated fats. Monounsaturated fat is a slightly un-saturated fat and polyunsaturated fat is a highly unsaturated fat. When substituted for saturated fat, both of these fats help reduce blood cholesterol.

Triglycerides   Triglycerides are another type of fat found in blood and food. Triglycerides in food are made up of both saturated and unsaturated fats. The liver also produces triglycerides; when excess calories and alcohol are consumed, the liver produces even more triglycerides. Elevated triglyceride levels are often seen when HDL is low and LDL is high. Lowering triglycerides can raise the good HDL. Very high levels of triglycerides can cause an inflammation of the pancreas (pancreatitis).

Sugar and Triglycerides Some individuals with elevated triglycerides are sensitive to sugar. When a high sugar diet is consumed, the pancreas responds by releasing too much insulin which acts to break down the sugar. This process results in a higher level of triglycerides. Decreasing sugar intake will usually lower triglyceride levels, but the beneficial effects seem to be greater for men than women.

Smoking
Smoking by women in this country causes almost as many deaths from heart disease as from lung cancer. Smokers are two to six times more likely to suffer a heart attack than non-smoking woman, and the risk increases with the number of cigarettes smoked each day. The risk of stroke is also increased in smokers as is the risk for cancers of the mouth, throat, lung, urinary tract, pancreas, and cervix as well as lung problems such as bronchitis and emphysema.

High Blood Pressure (Hypertension)
High blood pressure greatly increases the chances of developing cardiovascular disease. Stroke is a result of high blood pressure; even slightly high levels double your risk. Blood pressure tends to rise with age, and more than half of American women over age 55 have high blood pressure. Blood pressure is measured in millimeters (mm) of mercury (Hg); a level that stays above 140/90 mm Hg is considered to be high blood pressure. High blood pressure, frequently called hypertension, is often called the "silent killer" since most people can't tell they have it. Because hypertension can exist without warning, blood pressure should be checked regularly. Black women develop high blood pressure more often and more severely

than White women. No cure exists for high blood pressure, but it can be controlled. See Table 4-2.

Table 4-2
Blood Pressure Categories in Adults
(18 years and Older)

Blood pressure is shown as two numbers—the systolic pressure as the heart is beating and the diastolic pressure between heart beats. Both numbers are important.

Category	Blood Pressure Level in mm Hg Systolic	Diastolic
Normal	<130	<85
High Normal	130–139	85–89
Hypertension		
Stage 1	140–159	90–99
Stage 2	160–179	100–109
Stage 3	180–209	110–119
Stage 4	≥210	≥120

From The Fifth Report of the Joint National Committee on Detection, Evaluation,and Treatment of High Blood Pressure, NIH, NHLBI, 1993.

PREVENTION

The prevention of heart disease can begin at any time, but the smart practice is to start with children. For children, exercise, proper diet, and healthy habits should be introduced early in life. Children who are taught that health is a result of exercise and proper diet are more apt to develop health habits that will keep them fit. Knowing health is a matter of cause-and-effect does not always affect teenagers who often consider themselves to be immortal. Adolescents need to be reminded of the health lessons they learned when they were younger. Every adult can confirm that keeping tabs on your health is far easier than letting it get out of control. Seeking the advice of a health professional can help determine if any risk factors for cardiovascular disease exist for you. Even if you don't have any risk factors for cardiovascular disease, discussing preventive measures now, may lessen your chances of developing cardiovascular disease later.

The bottom line for heart health is not the health professional, but each woman, because you and only you can make the kind of lifestyle changes—changes in eating, smoking, and exercise—that will help protect against cardiovascular disease. In the meantime, keep reading.

Lowering Or Maintaining Blood Cholesterol Levels

Even those of you who may have no concerns about elevated cholesterol levels should listen to this advice since more than likely you will experience an increase in cholesterol levels once your estrogen levels begin to drop. This advice however does not apply to pregnant or nursing women and to children.

Positive Action   Reducing your blood cholesterol can greatly decrease the chances of developing coronary heart disease. For most people, total blood cholesterol and LDL cholesterol can be lowered by eating

- less saturated fat
- less total fat
- less cholesterol

Lowering LDL cholesterol is the main goal of treatment. Cutting down on fat intake also decreases calorie intake and leads to weight reduction which is another plus for heart health. Losing extra weight and becoming more physically active, as well as quitting smoking, may help boost HDL cholesterol levels. The need for cholesterol-lowering medications will depend on how high the LDL cholesterol level remains after positive changes have been made in diet and lifestyle. Risk factors for coronary heart disease are also considered.

Maximum Intake Levels   Total fat in the diet should not exceed 30% of the total calories taken in daily, and saturated fat should be no more than 10% of that. Learn to calculate the percentage of calories from fat in foods so that wise food choices can be made. Know that cholesterol intake should be less than 300 mg per day. See Table 4-3 "Figuring Out Fat" to determine your total fat intake.

Table 4-3
Figuring out Fat

Total Calories (per day)	Total Fat (in grams)	Saturated Fat (in grams)
1,200	40 or less (360 calories/or less)	13 or less (120 calories/or less)
1,400	47 or less (420 calories/or less)	16 or less (140 calories/or less)
1,600	53 or less (480 calories/or less)	18 or less (160 calories/or less)
2,000	67 or less (600 calories/or less)	22 or less (200 calories/or less)
2,400	80 or less (720 calories/or less	27 or less (240 calories/or less)

Total number of calories X 30% = total fat calories—divided by 9 gm = total number of fat grams; total number of calories X 10% = total saturated fat calories—divided by 9 gm = total number of saturated fat grams.

Dietary Guidelines   The National Heart, Lung, and Blood Institute from the National Institutes of Health recommends this eating pattern for all healthy Americans ages two and over, and especially for those who want to lower their blood cholesterol levels. Use Table 4-4 "A Guide to Low Fat, Low Cholesterol Foods" to choose low-saturated fat, low-cholesterol foods. If you follow this diet for 3 to 6 months and your blood cholesterol does not drop to a normal level, you may need to cut back still more on saturated fat and cholesterol.

To lower triglycerides and increase the good HDL

- limit alcohol intake to $1^{1}/_{2}$ – 2 ounces per day
- exercise regularly
- lose weight if overweight
- don't smoke
- no more than $^{1}/_{3}$ of the daily calories should come from fat (see Table 4-4 to help with food selection and cooking)

Table 4-4
A Guide to Choosing Low-Fat Low Cholesterol Foods

MEAT, POULTRY, FISH & SHELL FISH (up to 6 oz/day)

Choose	**Lean cuts of meat with fat trimmed, like:** • beef-round, sirloin, chuck, loin lamb-leg, arm, loin, rib • pork tenderloin, leg (fresh), shoulder (arm or picnic) • veal-all trimmed cuts except ground • poultry without skin • fish, shellfish
Decrease	**"Prime" grade fatty cuts of meat like:** • beef-corned, beef brisket, regular ground, short ribs • pork-spareribs, blade roll **Goose, domestic duck** **Organ meats, like liver, kidney, sweetbreads, brain** **Sausage, bacon, frankfurters,** **Regular luncheon meats** **Caviar, roe**

DAIRY PRODUCTS
(2 servings a day; 3 servings for women who are pregnant or breast feeding)

Choose	Skim milk, 1% milk, low-fat buttermilk, low-fat evaporated or nonfat milk Low-fat yogurt and low-fat frozen yogurt Low-fat soft cheeses, like: cottage, farmer, pot Cheese labeled no more than 2 to 6 grams of fat an ounce
Go Easy On!	2% milk Part-skim ricotta Part-skim or imitation hard cheeses like: part-skim mozzarella "Light" cream cheese "Light" sour cream
Decrease	Whole milk, like: regular, evaporated, condensed Cream, half-and-half, most nondairy creamers and products, real or nondairy whipped cream Cream cheese, sour cream, ice cream, custard-style yogurt Whole-milk ricotta High-fat cheese like: Neufchatel, Brie, Swiss, American, mozzarella, feta, cheddar, Muenster

EGGS (no more than 3 egg yolks/wk)

Choose	Egg whites Cholesterol- free egg substitutes
Decrease	Egg yolks

FRUITS& VEGETABLES
(2 to 4 servings of fruit and 3 to 5 servings of vegetables)

Choose	Fresh, frozen, canned, or dried fruits and vegetables
Decrease	Vegetables prepared in butter, cream, or sauce

Table 4-4 (continued)
A Guide to Choosing Low-Fat Low Cholesterol Foods

FAT & OILS (up to 6 to 8 tsp a day)

Choose
Unsaturated vegetable oils like: corn, olive, peanut, rapeseed (canola oil), safflower, sesame, soybean
Margarine or shortening made with unsaturated fats above: liquid tub, stick
Diet mayonnaise, salad dressings made with unsaturated fats listed above
Low-fat dressings

Go Easy On!
Nuts and seeds
Avocados and olives

Decrease
Butter, coconut oil, palm kernel oil, palm oil, lard, bacon fat
Margarine or shortening made with saturated fats listed above
Dressings made with egg yolk

BREADS, CEREALS, PASTA, RICE, DRIED PEAS, & BEANS
(6 to 11 servings a day)

Choose
Breads, like: white, whole wheat, pumpernickel, and rye breads; sandwich buns; dinner rolls; rice cakes
Low-fat crackers, like: matzo, pita; bagels, English muffins; bread sticks, rye krisp, saltines, zwieback
Hot cereals, most cold dry cereals
Pasta, like: plain noodles, spaghetti, macaroni
Any grain rice
Dried peas, and beans, like: split peas, black-eyed peas, chick peas, kidney beans, navy beans, lentils, soybeans, soybean curd (tofu)

Go Easy On!
Store-bought pancakes, waffles, biscuits, muffins, corn bread

Decrease
Croissants, butter rolls, sweet rolls, Danish pastry, doughnuts
Most snack crackers like: cheese crackers, butter crackers, those made with saturated fats
Granola-type cereals made with saturated fats
Pasta and rice prepared with cream, butter, or cheese sauces, egg noodles

SWEETS AND SNACKS (Avoid too many sweets)

Choose
Low-fat frozen desserts, like: sherbet, sorbet, italian ice, frozen yogurt, popsicles
Low-fat cakes, like: angel food cake
Low-fat cookies, like fig bars, gingersnaps
Low-fat candy, like: jelly beans, hard candy
Low-fat snacks, like: plain popcorn, pretzels
Nonfat beverages, like: carbonated drinks, juices, teas, coffee

Table 4-4 (continued)
A Guide to Choosing Low-Fat Low Cholesterol Foods

Go Easy On!	Frozen desserts, like: ice milk,
	Homemade cakes, cookies, and pies using unsaturated oils
	    sparingly
	Fruit crisps and cobblers
	Potato and corn chips prepared with unsaturated
	    vegetable oil

Decrease	High-fat frozen desserts like: ice cream, frozen tofu High-fat cakes, like: most store bought, pound, and frosted cakes Store-bought pies, most store-bought cookies Most candy, like: chocolate bars Potato and corn chips prepared with saturated fat Buttered popcorn High-fat beverages, like: frappes, milkshakes, floats, eggnogs

LABEL INGREDIENTS (To avoid much fat, saturated fat or cholesterol, go easy on products that list first any fat, oil, or ingredients higher in saturated fat or cholesterol. Choose more often those products that contain ingredients lower in saturated fat or cholesterol.)

Choose	Ingredients low in saturated fat or cholesterol: carob, cocoa Oils, like: corn, cottonseed, olive, safflower, sesame, soybean, sunflower Nonfat dry milk, nonfat dry milk solids, skim milk

Decrease	Ingredients high in saturated fat or cholesterol:
	Chocolate
	Animal fat, like: bacon, beef, ham, lamb, pork, chicken, or
	    turkey fats, butter, lard
	Coconut, coconut oil, palm-kernel or palm oil
	Cream
	Egg and egg-yolk solids
	Hardened fat or oil
	Hydrogenated vegetable oil
	Shortening or vegetable shortening, unspecified vegetable oil
	    (could be coconut, palm-kernel, palm)

Source: *The Healthy Heart Handbook for Women.* (1992). National Institutes of Health, National Heart, Lung and Blood Institute. Adapted from *Report of the Expert Panel on Detection, Evaluation, and Treatment of High Blood Cholesterol in Adults,* NHLBI, 1989. U.S. Department of Health and Human Services. NIH Publication No. 92-2720

Menu Planning Tips

Cholesterol Reduction Cooking.[4] Select fish, poultry, and lean cuts of meat, and remove fat from meats and skin from chicken. Fish and shell fish, in general, have a lot less saturated fat and cholesterol than meat and poultry. However, some shell fish is relatively high in cholesterol and should be eaten less often. High-fat fish, like salmon, rainbow trout, carp, herring, tuna and mackerel contain large amounts of omega-3 fatty acids. These fatty acids are effective in lowering blood triglycerides. Controversy exists as to whether they reduce blood cholesterol. The regular use of fish in the diet, however, is encouraged because it is low in saturated fat. The American Heart Association and many other health authorities do not recommend the use of fish oil supplements because their effectiveness and safety have not been adequately evaluated. Fish oils should not be self-prescribed. They are potent substances. See Table 4-5 for fish and shellfish comparison chart.

Table 4-5
Fish & Shellfish Omega-3 Fatty Acids, Fat & Cholesterol Content

Product (3½ oz. Cooked)	Saturated (Grams)	Cholesterol mg	Omega-3 Fatty acids (Grams)	Total Fat (Grams)	Total Calories
Finfish					
Haddock	0.2	74	0.2	0.9	112
Cod	0.2	55	0.2	0.9	105
Pollock	0.2	96	1.5	1.1	113
Perch	0.2	42	0.3	1.2	117
Grouper	0.3	47	---	1.3	118
Whiting	0.3	84	0.9	1.7	115
Snapper	0.4	47	---	1.7	128
Halibut	0.4	41	0.6	2.9	140
Rockfish	0.5	44	0.5	2.0	121
Sea Bass	0.7	53	---	2.5	124
Trout	0.8	73	0.9	4.3	151
Swordfish	1.4	50	1.1	5.1	155
Tuna	1.6	49	---	6.3	184
Salmon	1.9	87	1.3	11.0	216
Anchovy	2.2	---	2.1	9.7	210
Herring	2.6	77	2.1	11.5	203
Mackerel	4.2	75	1.3	17.8	262
Pompano	4.5	64	---	12.1	211
Crustaceans					
Lobster	0.1	72	0.1	0.6	98
Crab, blue	0.2	100	0.5	1.8	102
Shrimp	0.3	195	0.3	1.1	99
Mollusks					
Clams	0.2	67	0.3	2.0	148
Mussel	0.9	56	0.8	4.5	172
Oyster	1.3	109	1.0	5.0	137

U.S. Department of Health and Human Services. NIH Publication No. 92-2920.
--- = Information not available in sources used

- Broil, bake, roast, or poach foods rather than fry them.

- Reduce the amount of sausage, bacon, and processed high-fat cold cuts.

- Limit organ meats such as liver, kidney, or brains

- Use low-fat alternatives. Drink skim, low-fat, or reconstituted nonfat dry milk in place of whole milk. Use low-fat yogurt, buttermilk, or evaporated skim milk in place of cream or sour cream. Use low-fat cheeses. Sherbet or low-fat frozen yogurt can be a delicious replacement for ice cream. The selection of non-fat yogurt, ice cream, and cheeses is becoming more prevalent.

- Use margarine or liquid vegetable oils high in unsaturated fats in place of butter. However, all fats and oils should be used sparingly.

- Eat egg yolks in moderation. Egg whites contain no fat or cholesterol and may be eaten often. They also can be used in most recipes that call for eggs.

- Fruits, vegetables, cereals, breads, rice, and pasta made from whole grains are good sources of starch and fiber, and usually contain no cholesterol and little or no saturated fat.

- Small amounts of liquid vegetable oils are a good choice for sauteing vegetables, browning potatoes, popping corn; and for making baked goods, pancakes, and waffles.

- Substitute unsaturated fats (polyunsaturated and monounsaturated) for saturated fat since unsaturated fat actually helps to lower cholesterol levels. Polyunsaturated fats are found primarily in safflower, corn, soybean, cottonseed, sesame, and sunflower oils, which are common cooking oils. Polyunsaturated fats are contained in most salad dressings. But be cautious— commercially prepared salad dressings also may be high in saturated fats, and therefore careful inspection of labels is important. The word "hydrogenated" on a label means that some of the polyunsaturated fat has been converted to saturated fat. Monounsaturated fats are found primarily in olive and canola oil. Like other vegetable oils, these oils are used in cooking as well as in salads.

- Many store-bought baked goods, snacks, and other pre-pared foods have hidden saturated fats; because they are made with lard, butter, cream, coconut oil, or palm oil. Develop a habit of reading the product labels. New food labeling on all processed foods, meat, and poultry items lists total calories, calories from fat, total fat, saturated fat, and cholesterol in addition to other nutrients. Choose a product with the lowest proportion of saturated fat. The label also tells you something else about a product. Ingredients are listed in order of amount from most to least by weight. So, when you buy a breakfast cereal, for example, choose one that has a whole grain listed first (such as whole wheat or oatmeal). Many bakery items are now available which contain no cholesterol or fat, but beware since they are often high in calories.

- Be aware of the sources of fat—especially hidden fat—in your diet. For example, some crackers and cereals are high in fat.

- Do not be misled by the NO ANIMAL FAT OR LOW OR NO CHOLESTEROL label on some foods. A fat can have no cholesterol but still be highly saturated if it contains coconut oil, palm oil, palm-kernel oil, chocolate, or hydrogenated vegetable oils. These items may still contain a large amount of fat or saturated fat. Examples are peanut butter, solid vegetable shortening, nondairy creamer, and baked products like cookies, cakes, and crackers. For people trying to lose excess weight or reduce their blood cholesterol level, these foods should be chosen less often.

- A variety of lower-fat products have been introduced during the past few years which has made it much easier to control our fat intake. These include meats, dairy products, and processed foods. Fat-free salad dressings, crackers, and snack foods are appearing on grocery shelves in greater quantities. Food manufacturers are formulating their products using the lowest amount and least-saturated oils possible to achieve quality and taste.

- A lifelong commitment to sensible eating and exercise is required to lead a heart-healthy lifestyle.

Cholesterol Reduction And Fiber
Although reducing the intake of saturated fat and cholesterol

is usually the first step in the management of high cholesterol levels, these efforts may not reduce cholesterol to acceptable levels. A water-soluble fiber, psyllium hydrophilic mucilloid, has been found to be capable of reducing both total and LDL cholesterol levels by 5 to 8% in mild to moderate increased cholesterol levels. This product is better known as "a natural vegetable laxative" or psyllium fiber that is a bulk forming laxative which increases the bulk of the stool. Psyllium is a natural soluble fiber derived from the husk of the blond psyllium seeds.

The mechanisms by which soluble fibers reduce total and LDL cholesterol levels are unknown, but psyllium hydrophilic mucilloid appears to be a safe and effective means to increase soluble fiber intake and reduce blood cholesterol levels. To be effective, approximately 10.2 grams or 3 rounded teaspoons taken daily are combined with a low-cholesterol, low-fat diet. This relatively simple fiber is without significant side effects and has been shown to provide a continuous cholesterol-lowering effect for up to 4 months or longer if it is continued.[7,8] Eating a variety of fruits and vegetables, legumes, and oat bran is another way to increase fiber intake.

How Do I Put It All Together?

Trying to plan a low-fat, low-cholesterol diet may appear complex; if you are also trying to maintain a high calcium intake to prevent osteoporosis, the task may seem very complicated. Fear not, meal planning becomes much easier once a person knows which foods to consume. Dietary aids are available to ease the process. Table 4-4 will guide you through the selection process, and the menu planning tips in the previous pages should make this a relatively easy task.

Controlling Blood Pressure

According to the National Heart, Lung, and Blood Institute at the National Institutes of Health, high blood pressure can be controlled with proper treatment. If you don't have high blood pressure now, you can take steps to prevent it from developing. Control and prevention of high blood pressure can begin with the following actions.

- If you are overweight, lose weight

- If you drink alcohol, no more than 12 ounces of beer, 5 ounces of wine, or 1$^{1}/_{2}$ ounces of hard liquor should be consumed daily

- Exercise regularly. Regular aerobic exercise such as brisk walking, bicycling, jogging, or swimming helps control weight, benefits the entire cardiovascular system, and contributes to bone health as well.

- Try to use as little salt as possible both in cooking and at the table. Remember, salt is hidden in many foods such as lunch meat, cured meats, cheese, canned vegetables and soups, frozen dinners, prepared snacks, and condiments such as catsup, soy sauce, pickles, and olives. Fortunately several products are currently available that are "no sodium" or "low sodium." Check product labels for the amount of sodium in each serving. Many experts advise a total daily salt intake of no more than 6 grams which equals about 2400 milligrams of sodium— this includes whatever is added during cooking and at the table.

- Beware of salt substitutes with potassium chloride since they can be harmful to people affected with certain medical problems. Seek the advice of your health professional before using salt substitutes.

- Most importantly make certain you take any medication that is prescribed as directed. If any of your medications cause you to "feel different," consult your health professional, and DO NOT discontinue it unless your health professional has advised you to do so.

Kicking The Smoking Habit

No Such Thing As No Risk Smoking   Do not be misled by advertising that leads you to believe some cigarettes are of lower risk than others. There is just no safe way to smoke! Low-tar and low-nicotine cigarettes may reduce the risk of lung cancer, but they do not lessen the risks of heart disease. Not smoking at all is the only safe and healthy way "to smoke."

Quitting Hundreds of methods exist to help a person stop smoking. The most effective method involves personal determination and just "quitting." If you have tried and failed, don't give up. Know that there are as many ex-smokers in this country as there are smokers. You can stop and don't let anyone, including yourself, tell you otherwise. Although giving up cigarettes is not an easy task, the result of good health is worth the struggle. Not only are the risks of heart disease substantially decreased, even to the point where the risk is the same as if you had never smoked, but you will also feel better. Just ask any ex-smoker. Other benefits of being an ex-smoker exist. You will

- lessen your chances of getting lung cancer, emphysema, and other lung diseases
- have fewer colds or flu
- smell better—your clothes, home, car, and breath
- no longer be breathless after climbing stairs and walking
- lose that morning cough
- have fewer wrinkles
- stop subjecting the people around you to second-hand smoke, thereby, possibly decreasing their upper respiratory problems
- have more energy
- feel good about the accomplishment achieved and the control you now have over your life

OTHER RISK PREVENTION ACTIVITIES

Losing Weight

Body Shape If you are overweight, losing pounds can lower the chances of developing cardiovascular disease. While being overweight raises your risk for heart disease, body shape may affect heart health as well. "Apple-shaped" individuals with extra fat at the waistline may have a higher risk than "pear-shaped" people with heavy hips and thighs. If your waist is nearly as large or larger than the size of your hips, a higher risk for coronary heart disease exists.

Diabetes Weight loss reduces the risk of developing diabetes—a serious condition that raises the risk of coronary heart disease. More than 80% of people who have diabetes die of some type of cardiovascular disease, usually heart attack. Compared with non diabetic women, diabetic women are also more apt to suffer from high blood pressure and high blood cholesterol.

Healthy Outcome Shedding pounds lowers high blood pressure and cholesterol. In fact, if blood pressure and cholesterol are only slightly or moderately high, weight loss may be the only treatment needed. Furthermore, if medication for high blood pressure or elevated cholesterol levels is required, the lower your weight, the less medication you may need.

Formula For Success To lose weight, take in fewer calories than you burn. So either reduce the number of calories consumed, or increase your activity level. An ideal strategy would include doing both. See Chapter 6 for strategies for a weight reduction program.

Physical Activity
Physical inactivity has become recognized as an important risk factor for heart disease, both as a risk factor alone and as one that influences other risk factors such as high blood pressure, high blood cholesterol, and obesity. Regular physical activity will help reduce the risk of coronary heart disease.

Physical activity does not need to be intense to be beneficial. Even low- to moderate-intensity activity can help lower the risk of heart disease. Examples of such activity are pleasure walking, stair climbing, gardening, yard work, moderate-to-heavy housework, dancing, and home exercise. To get heart benefits from these activities, do one or more of them every day. More vigorous exercise improves the fitness of the heart which can lower heart disease risk even more. "Aerobic" exercise which includes brisk walking, jogging, cycling, jumping rope, cross-country skiing, and swimming 30 minutes a day, three or four times a week, strengthens your heart and lungs.[9]

Exercise helps take off extra pounds, controls blood pressure, lessens a diabetic's need for insulin, and may boost the level of "good" HDL-cholesterol. Choose an activity that fits your schedule and lifestyle. BEFORE YOU START AN EXERCISE PROGRAM CONSULT YOUR HEALTH CARE PROFESSIONAL, especially if you have not been used to energetic activity. See Chapter 6 and Appendix A for more heart and bone exercise activities.

Hormones

Hormone Replacement Therapy   Should menopausal and postmenopausal women use "hormone replacement therapy" to prevent heart disease? This is a hot topic in the field of menopause today. And again no simple answer to this question exists. For some postmenopausal women, hormone replacement therapy has been the treatment of choice to help replace the estrogen lost due to menopause. Hormone replacement therapy has been recognized for its cardiovascular benefits, mainly due to the positive effect of estrogen on cholesterol or blood lipids.

Estrogen   Estrogen taken alone lowers the low-density lipids (LDL) and raises high-density lipids (HDL) cholesterol. New studies are now telling us estrogen does more than just affect the blood lipids. Estrogen seems to also have an effect on the lining of the blood vessels so that plaque or fatty deposits are not laid down as easily. Estrogen may also play a role in increasing coronary blood flow and possibly dilating the coronary arteries. Furthermore, it keeps the blood "thin" so it doesn't coagulate or clot easily. All of these conditions play a major part in heart attack and heart disease. Many studies have shown a 50% reduction in heart disease risk in postmenopausal women taking estrogen.

Estrogen And Progesterone   While the benefits of estrogen are being discovered, less is known about the effects of combined estrogen and progesterone. Progesterone is usually given to women to protect the lining of the uterus. There are, however, reports of possible negative effects of progesterone on blood lipids which indicate that progesterone may reverse or blunt the positive action of estrogen. However, the results of a recent study have shown otherwise. The study compared women who have taken no estrogen, estrogen alone, or estrogen and progesterone together. Women on estrogen or estrogen and progesterone had lower rates for a first heart attack and better heart attack survival rates than non-users (women not on estrogen or estrogen and progesterone). Even better results were reported for those who were on the combination of estrogen and progesterone.

Best Bet   Despite the controversies and lack of what some might call good clinical research, the American College of Physicians concludes that women "who have coronary heart disease or who are at increased risk for coronary artery disease are likely to benefit from hormone therapy." And according to one well known expert in the field of cardiovascular disease, "that is sound advice."[10,11,12]

For those women at risk for cardiovascular disease, the evidence available thus far seems to show hormone replacement therapy is a logical decision. For those who choose not to or cannot take hormones, elimination of all possible risk factors plus aggressive dietary and exercise programs are the next best thing. For a greater in depth look at types and combinations and pros and cons of hormones see Chapter 5.

Diet, Weight Loss, Exercise—Men And Women

For reasons that are unclear, women do not respond as favorably as men to diet, weight loss, and exercise in altering lipid levels. Studies show low-fat diets do not work as well in postmenopausal women as they do in men. Exercise raises HDL and lowers LDL levels better in men than women. In the area of exercise, research studies on women have often raised more questions. The information gathered on duration and intensity of exercise is sometimes not clear, and in some studies cigarette smoking, alcohol use, diet, and use of hormones has not been reported. In spite of all of this, enough reliable evidence has been gathered and continues to be gathered to show that alterations in blood lipids are beneficial in preventing coronary artery disease in women as well as in men. All studies on both men and women with severe cases of elevated cholesterol levels do agree that an aggressive program to lower LDL and raise HDL stops the progression of heart disease in both sexes.

The Aspirin Question

You may have heard that taking aspirin regularly can help prevent heart attacks. Is this a good idea for you? The role of aspirin in the prevention of cardiovascular disease has been the focus of considerable research, especially in men where studies have shown that aspirin can help prevent heart attacks. However, a fairly recent study of more than 87,000 women, the first to suggest a similar benefit for women, found that women who took a low dose of aspirin regularly were less likely to suffer a first heart attack than women who took no aspirin. Older women appeared to benefit the most.[13]

While these reports are encouraging, more study is needed before we can be sure that aspirin is safe and effective in preventing heart attacks in women. What is known for sure is that you should not take aspirin to prevent a heart attack without first discussing it with your health professional. Aspirin is a powerful drug with many side effects. It can increase your chances of getting ulcers and suffering a stroke from a hemorrhage.[4]

FOR MORE INFORMATION

If you want to know more about keeping your heart healthy, the National Heart, Lung, and Blood Institute located at the National Institutes of Health has fact sheets on preventing high blood pressure, preventing high blood cholesterol, the heart benefits of physical activity, and heart disease risk factors for women. See "Resources" section at the end of this book for further information.

Chapter Five

How to Manage it All

Areoccurring theme has now developed. Women experience menopause either naturally or artificially through surgery. Menopause brings a reduction in the production of estrogen. Further, an estrogen deficiency is associated with the development of osteoporosis, cardiovascular changes, hot flashes, insomnia, depression, sexual difficulties, and urinary problems.

If a lack of the hormone estrogen supposedly causes problems, then why not just replace it? This simple solution is actually the basis of hormone replacement therapy (HRT) which many health care providers prescribe today. Yet hormone replacement therapy is not a simple answer as all the current controversy proves. Many questions are outstanding.

- How much estrogen should be replaced?
- How should the estrogen be administered?
- Should the estrogen be naturally produced, or are chemically manufactured (synthetic) products all right?
- What are the side effects of estrogen?
- Should estrogen be given alone?
- What form of estrogen is best?
- How long should estrogen be given—months, years, forever?
- Is there an alternative to hormone replacement?

Prepare for a "rocky road" of decision making since the path, though clear in many respects, is full of detours and confusing landmarks. Each question usually has many possible answers. Often, deciding to proceed with hormone replacement therapy entails a benefit/risk analysis—does the benefit of the therapy outweigh other possible health hazards? We make benefit/risk decisions every day. Trying to decide how to reach a particular destination is an example of a benefit/risk analysis. Is it better to take an airplane or an automobile? Both alternatives will provide benefits and risks. You measure the benefits against the risks posed by each method of transportation and then decide which is best for you. Avoiding benefit/risk decisions is a poor solution. In the case of the transportation decision, avoidance would leave you sitting at home.

Fortunately, no woman must make her decisions alone. Her health care provider will supply her with answers to her questions, but an informed woman will ask better questions. The following chapter will provide any woman a solid basis to ask relevant questions. Look for a review of estrogen and progesterone, a discussion of types of estrogen and progesterone administration, an overview of administration schedules, suggestions for women who cannot take estrogen; and the reasons for and against estrogen usage.

HORMONE REPLACEMENT THERAPY— NOT A WHIM

The advantages of using hormones to control menopausal symptoms have been known for over 60 years. The 1940s saw a link established between a lack of estrogen in the body and osteoporosis. In the 1950s, the medical community recognized that estrogen had an effect on cardiovascular disease. Recognition of the importance of estrogen continued in the 1960s and 1970s as other short-term benefits of estrogen became apparent, and estrogen replacement therapy became very popular. Prescriptions more than doubled during this period. Sales dropped sharply when the increased risk of uterine cancer, with use of estrogen alone, became apparent. But since the 1970s when the use of progesterone, in addition to estrogen, was found to not only reduce, but sharply decrease, the incidence of uterine cancer, the use of estrogen increased and has continued to increase.[1]

Before continuing the discussion of hormone replacement therapy, a brief review of estrogen and its various forms is warranted.

Estrogen

Estrogens are the hormones mainly responsible for female sex characteristics. Estrogen production occurs primarily in the female ovary, but fat cells are also responsible for some level of production. Producing estrogen is not specific to females, men also produce low levels of estrogen in the testes. When menopause occurs, either naturally or artificially by way of surgery, radiation, or chemotherapy, specific hormones become deficient, most importantly, estrogen in the form of 17B-estradiol and progesterone. Before menopause, the predominant form of estrogen is estradiol—a naturally occurring estrogen produced primarily by the ovary.

Estrone Before menopause a second major form of estrogen is produced in the form of estrone. Estrone, like estradiol, is naturally produced but is not as potent as estradiol. After menopause estrone becomes the predominant form of estrogen and most of it is made in fatty tissue. After a natural menopause, a very small amount of estradiol may still be produced by the ovaries, but most of the limited supply of estradiol will now come from estrone.

Estriol Another natural human estrogen is estriol which is only produced in any significant amount during pregnancy. In the nonpregnant state, its importance is questionable. Considered a weak estrogen, estriol can be used to treat hot flashes and manage vaginal dryness, but it plays no part in preventing osteoporosis. While its use against vaginal dryness is limited, estriol may be suggested for use by women who cannot take estrogen by mouth, skin patch, or injection. Further studies are required before any definite recommendations can be made.

The Value Of Hormone Replacement Therapy

Although enthusiasm for the use of postmenopausal hormone replacement therapy has wavered over the past four decades, qualified evidence does exist that for some the use of hormone replacement therapy may be a key factor in keeping women alive and healthy. Although the Food and Drug Administration (FDA) has approved the use of estrogen replacement therapy for prevention of osteoporosis, the same approval for its use in the prevention and treatment of heart disease has not yet been given.

HOW TO DECIDE ABOUT HRT

The Controversy

Medical studies are very time-consuming and complex. Research data is thoroughly reviewed before full approval is granted for any treatment program. This cautious environment affects the full approval of hormone replacement therapy. Whereas an idea like hormone replacement therapy may be accepted, the way the hormones are taken—by pill or cream or injection—may not be. Current evidence supports the notion that estrogen replacement therapy protects postmenopausal women against coronary artery disease, but the best type and length of treatment remains controversial. Some of the reasons the use of estrogen replacement therapy has not been accepted completely have to do with the way the studies were conducted and the absence of certain kinds of information. For example, in some of the studies, details about the type or dose of estrogen or how long it was used are unclear.

Studies Are Long Time also affects the acceptance of some treatment options; time is needed to study the effects of new therapies. The routine addition of progestins to prevent estrogen-induced uterine cancer did not occur until the 1970s, hence the limited research information on this combined form of treatment.

Hormones Are Complex Hormones are not just simple chemicals. They can perform not just one but many functions in the body at the same time. These multiple actions can cause some confusion when discussing hormone replacement therapy. Progestins for example may help to prevent estrogen-induced uterine cancer and may increase the action of estrogen on bone, but have been reported to counteract the benefits of estrogen on coronary disease. Report of a new study, although limited in scope, which appears later in this chapter has found otherwise. Whether progestin has a protective effect on the breast has not yet been firmly established. Even prolonged use of estrogen as a causative agent of breast cancer has been questioned, although many studies seem to indicate the risks are low.

A Personal Decision   In the face of conflicting and inconclusive studies, the decision to take hormone replacement therapy is a personal one to be decided by each woman in consultation with her health care professional. The decision whether or not to take HRT may be the most complex medical decision that any woman will face in her lifetime. According to several experts who have studied estrogen and progestin replacement therapy for some time, the majority of evidence is reassuring, but for some women the risks may outweigh the benefits, and this is a decision that only she and her health care provider together can make.

Once Decided, Then What Kind?   Once the decision has been made to use hormone replacement therapy (HRT), the next issue is to decide what kind should be used. Many options are available. Many effective estrogen preparations differ in their potency, origin, length of action, and cost. It is also important to know that individual women differ in their response to different kinds of hormones as well as the dose and schedule. Which essentially means is that not all women are treated exactly the same! Hormone replacement therapy is not like treating a "strep" throat, when most adults, with the exception of those with an allergy to the medication, are usually treated with similar doses of penicillin. Oral estrogens, primarily Premarin, have been available for over 50 years and most of the long-term benefits of estrogen are based on experience with oral use.

TYPES OF ESTROGEN

Oral Estrogens

Oral estrogens have been available for over 50 years. Natural estrogens are preferred for estrogen replacement therapy, because they are not as strong as the synthetic estrogens used in the contraceptive pill. Synthetic (artificially produced) estrogens are very different from natural estrogen and are between 100 and 1000 times stronger than their natural counterparts.

In the United States, conjugated equine estrogens (CEE) are the most commonly prescribed estrogens for hormone replacement therapy. These estrogens are obtained from the urine of pregnant horses.

Premarin® (Wyeth-Ayerst)—a mixture of estrogenic substances such as estrone, equilin, and smaller amounts of many other estrogens. Doses of oral CEE used today, such as 0.625 and 1.25 mg/day, mimic the lower levels of estradiol and estrone produced in a normal ovarian cycle. This preparation has been found to be effective in relieving menopausal symptoms and in the prevention of osteoporosis. Several studies have also found that it is effective in the prevention of cardiovascular disease in women. Two new products, Premphase™ and Prempro™, have been introduced which package the premarin tablets and the progestin tablets together for convenience. Just like Premarin, both products are indicated for the prevention of osteoporosis and alleviation of symptoms associated with menopause.

- **Premphase™**—contains both 0.625 mg of Premarin and progestin (5 mg of medroxyprogesterone acetate) tablets packaged together for a cyclic schedule. The Premarin is taken for 28 days and progestin from days 15 through 28.

- **Prempro™**—contains both a 0.625 mg tablet of
  Premarin and a progestin tablet (2.5 mg of medroxyprogesterone acetate) packaged together for consumption once a day for a continuous schedule.

Estrace (Bristol-Myers Squibb) Estradiol tablets—available in
doses ranging from 0.5 to 2 mg with a usual dose of 1 to 2 mg
daily. During absorption, the estradiol changes to estrone and
other estrogens before passage into the general circulation.
This preparation has been reported to be effective in relieving
menopausal symptoms and for the prevention of osteoporosis.

Ogen (Upjohn) Estropipate tablets—a form of estrone—a
dose of 0.625 mg will effectively relieve hot flashes and prevent osteoporosis.

Estratab (Solvay) Esterified estrogens tablets—principally
estrone— a dose of 0.3 mg to 2.5 mg/day has been reported to
be effective in relieving menopausal symptoms.

Menest (Smithkline Beecham) Esterified estrogens tablets—
principally estrone—a usual dose of 0.3 mg to 1.25 mg has been
reported to be effective in relieving menopausal symptoms.

Ortho-Est (Ortho) Estropipate tablets—a form of estrone—
a dose of 0.625 mg to 1.25 mg/day has been reported to be
effective in relieving menopausal symptoms.

Estratest (Solvay) Esterified estrogens and methyltestos-
terone—contains 0.625 mg of esterified estrogens and 1.25
mg of testosterone or 1.25 mg of esterified estrogens with 2.5
mg of testosterone, used to control menopausal symptoms
that are not improved by estrogen alone.

Oral administration of estrogen is safe and generally well tolerated. The dose can be adjusted easily and treatment can be
stopped immediately if necessary. Some individuals may experience nausea and others may have difficulty absorbing the
estrogen because of small bowel disease.

Nonoral Estrogens

Nonoral estrogens avoid passage through the gastrointestinal tract and the liver, often referred to in the medical literature as the "first pass effect" which is a complicated and incompletely understood process. What this essentially means is that by using preparations that are not initially exposed to the liver, problems and benefits associated with this first exposure such as increased blood pressure, clotting problems, and negative effects on the blood lipids do not occur.

Transdermal Patches   Developed in the early 1980s, transdermal patches (Estraderm) which were the first approved for clinical use in the United States, are designed to deliver estradiol daily through the skin into the bloodstream. Small quantities of the naturally occurring hormone estradiol are absorbed through the skin from the transdermal system, ensuring a continuous supply of circulating hormone in the body. Furthermore, when estradiol is administered through the skin, the drug does not undergo the rapid chemical changes in the liver and stomach that would occur if taken by mouth. Through regular use, Estraderm provides relief of the symptoms of menopause, has been shown to help prevent osteoporosis, and limited studies have even shown a positive effect on blood lipids.

The patches are applied to the skin, usually on the trunk of the body (including the buttocks and abdomen) and changed twice weekly. Although generally well tolerated, some patch users may develop skin reactions, the majority of which are mild. As with oral therapy, an adjustment of dosage is easily made, and treatment can be stopped immediately if required.

The FDA has approved two new estrogen patches for the treatment of moderate-to-severe menopause symptoms. One of the patches, Vivelle, is applied twice-weekly as is the Estraderm patch, but is smaller in size and available in four dosages. The other new transdermal system, Climara, is applied once-a-week.

Percutaneous (Through The Skin) The percutaneous administration of estradiol in an alcohol-based gel has been used for
estrogen replacement therapy in Europe but is not approved
for use in this country. The gel is applied to the arms, shoulders, and abdomen. The problem with estrogen replacement
of this kind is controlling the amount of estrogen the body
absorbs.

Vaginal Creams The lining of the vagina easily absorbs most
estrogen preparations such as vaginal tablets, vaginal rings,
and creams. At this time, only estrogen creams are available
since they are the only vaginal preparation approved in this
country. Vaginal creams are usually applied once or twice
weekly to limit problems associated with vaginal dryness,
sexual difficulties, and urinary problems. Although many
women will also notice an improvement in other symptoms
like hot flashes, these creams should only be used to soothe
vaginal problems, because the amount of estrogen being
absorbed cannot be accurately controlled. A progestin may
be prescribed for those women who use the vaginal cream on
a regular basis to prevent increased growth of the uterine lining. These creams should not be used in those women who
have reasons to avoid the use of estrogen.

Which Method Is Best?
No one answer can be given as to the best method of taking
estrogen. There is still much to be learned about each
method. The advantages and disadvantages of oral versus
nonoral estrogen methods and their effects upon various diseases such as high blood pressure and heart disease still are
not clear. It would be beneficial to know if oral estrogen
reduces heart disease risk or affects blood pressure more than
nonoral estrogens or vice versa, but as yet no proof exists to
support one method over another. What is known is that all
estrogens eventually end up in the blood which passes
through the liver every few minutes, so no matter how the
estrogen got into the body it will affect liver metabolism to
some degree.[2]

Summary Of Methods

- Synthetic estrogens such as ethinyl estradiol, the estrogen used in most oral contraceptives, are not recommended for postmenopausal women, because of the negative effects on the liver.

- Oral conjugated estrogens, estradiol, and estrone all have favorable or good effects on blood lipids, slow bone loss, and generally relieve the usual problems associated with menopause.

- Nonoral methods have a favorable effect on bone and with long-term use have shown favorable effects on the blood lipids. Thus, both oral and nonoral methods of treatment may equally protect the bones and cardiovascular system.

- Vaginal estrogen creams are best used with the oral preparations on a short-term basis. Continuous use of the vaginal creams, solely, is discouraged because of the difficulty in determining the amount absorbed into the system, especially for the woman with a uterus. The creams should be used if needed to take care of local problems of the vagina and urinary tract. See Table 5-1 for commonly used estrogen and progesterone preparations.

ANDROGEN

Androgens are the source of all estrogens in the body of men and women. The normal premenopausal ovary produces estrogen, progesterone, and androgen. The postmenopausal ovary produces androgen. The total postmenopausal levels of androgens are slightly lower than the premenopausal levels. After menopause or following a hysterectomy with removal of the ovaries, the adrenal gland bears the burden of androgen secretion.

The role of androgens in menopausal HRT is an area of great controversy. Many believe that adding androgens to treatment is dangerous, while others believe that androgens are key in maintaining premenopausal energy levels, intelligent thinking, and sex drive. There are, however, preparations of androgens and estrogen plus androgens available and although they have never gained widespread use in hormone replacement therapy, there have been positive reports of relief from hot flashes, increased sex drive, and a sense of well being.

Potential side effects of androgen therapy may be controlled with decreased doses and include:

- negative effects on blood lipids
- increased risk of breast cancer
- abnormal liver functions tests in those who take the oral preparations
- acne
- facial hair
- development of masculine-like tendencies
- increase in size of clitoris
- voice change
- psychological changes

A progesterone preparation is required for those women with a uterus on estrogen-androgen therapy just as in those taking estrogen without androgen. According to some experts, routine use of androgen in HRT should be avoided but may be helpful for unresolved symptoms of natural or surgical menopause in carefully selected women who do not respond to estrogen alone.[3,4]

Regarding androgens, the development of a wider body of knowledge about their use in hormone replacement therapy is needed.[3]

PROGESTERONE, PROGESTOGENS, PROGESTINS

In the premenopausal years, women produce progesterone which is responsible for the shedding of the uterine lining, whereas postmenopausal women produce very little. Postmenopausal women with an intact uterus, who receive estrogen therapy, have an increased incidence of excessive growth or thickening of the lining of the uterus. This increased growth may lead to cancer of the lining of the uterus. More than a decade of research has shown that the increased risk of uterine cancer is almost eliminated when estrogen therapy is combined with a progesterone which works to stop the growth of the uterine lining and reduces the risk of cancer of the uterus.

Progesterone can be taken in its native or natural form, or a synthetic or manufactured type may be used. Progesterone is the native form. Synthetic forms of progesterone are called progestogens or progestins. The terms progesterone, progestogens, and progestins are terms which are often used interchangeably, yet they are different.

Progesterone is produced by the ovary after ovulation. Progestins and progestogens are manufactured forms of the native hormone and have progesterone-like activity. Synthetic forms are necessary because

- natural progesterone is poorly absorbed by the body and is rapidly inactivated by the liver; may be given by injection to women who are unable to tolerate the synthetic forms.

- no transdermal or patch delivery system is available in the U.S.

- oral preparations of natural progesterone are currently not approved by the Food and Drug Administration.

Types Of Progestins

Two families of synthetic progestins exist—progesterone derivatives, medroxyprogesterone acetate (MPA) and megesterol acetate; and nortestosterone derivatives, norethindrone, norethindrone acetate, and norgestrel. Experts say the nortestosterone types tend to produce less bleeding (fewer days and lesser flow). Although all of these types act very much like progesterone, many differences exist in terms of how quickly they are absorbed by the body, how strong they are, and their side effects.[5,6] Adjusting the dosage or kind of progestin will alleviate problems such as midcycle bleeding.

How Progestins Work

Progestins actually protect the uterus by eliminating from the body any buildup of tissue from estrogen therapy. When this happens, bleeding comes from the uterus through the vagina similar to a menstrual period. This, however, is not a menstrual period since menstrual periods are related to ovulation. Ovulation no longer takes place in the postmenopausal woman, so pregnancy cannot occur. Furthermore this monthly bleeding is usually of a predictable nature, lasts a short length time, is of less quantity, and is not usually associated with cramping. This type of bleeding, known as "withdrawal bleeding" may continue in decreasing amounts until age 60 or longer. Any bleeding other than the planned bleeding from the progestin therapy should be reported to your health care provider.

The FDA has not yet issued an indication for the use of progestins in the prevention of uterine cancer. However, pharmaceutical companies are now suggesting in their "package inserts" that the addition of a progestin for 10 to 13 days for those on estrogen therapy has been found to afford protection against excess growth of the uterine lining.

TREATMENT SCHEDULES

Every woman has experienced the cyclic nature of the menstrual cycle. A woman can almost feel the changing hormone levels each month. This same cyclic process has been applied to the hormones used to treat the symptoms of menopause. Therefore, many of the treatments are prescribed on some type of schedule. Some treatment schedules have yet to be defined; for example, the optimal treatment schedule for estrogen plus progestin therapy has not been established. Two common schedules are described as cyclic and continuous. With cyclic schedules, therapy is taken for a specified period and then stopped for a specified length of time. In continuous therapy, there is no interruption or "time off." A

Table 5-1
Estrogen And Progesterone Preparations

	Dose	Manufacturer
Oral Estrogens		
Estrace	0.5 mg 1.0 mg 2.0 mg	Bristol-Myers Squibb
Estratab	0.3 mg 0.625 mg 1.25 mg 2.5 mg	Solvay
Estratest (combined estrogen & testosterone)	0.625\1.25 mg 1.25/2.5 mg	Solvay
Menest	0.3 mg 0.625 mg 1.25 mg 2.5 mg	SmithKline Beecham
Ogen	0.625 mg 1.25 mg 2.5 mg	Upjohn
Ortho-Est	0.625 mg 1.25 mg	Ortho
Premarin	0.3 mg 0.625 mg 0.9 mg 1.25 mg 2.5 mg	Wyeth-Ayerst
Premphase (combined estrogen & MPA*)	0.625/5 mg	Wyeth-Ayerst
Prempro (combined estrogen & MPA*)	0.625/2.5 mg	Wyeth-Ayerst

description of a variety of schedules can be found in Figure 5-1; even these schedules may have many variations:

Cyclic Estrogen Alone Or Unopposed Estrogen
Used prior to the 1970s, this treatment is not usually recommended for individuals with a uterus. This treatment resulted in excessive growth of the lining of the uterus which led to uterine cancer. Occasionally, this method is still used for the woman who has great difficulty tolerating progestin. If this is

Table 5-1 (continued)
Estrogen And Progesterone Preparations

	Dose	Manufacturer
Non-oral Estrogens		
Transdermal		
Estraderm	.05 mg	Ciba-Geigy
	0.1 mg	
Climara	.05 mg	Berlex
	0.1 mg	
Vaginal Creams		
Estrace	0.01 %	Bristol-Myers Squibb
Ogen	1.5 mg/gram	Upjohn
Ortho Dienestrol	0.01 %	Ortho
Premarin	0.625 mg/gram	Wyeth-Ayerst
Oral Progestins		
Aygestin (norethindrone acetate)	5 mg	ESI Pharma
Cycrin (MPA*)	2.5 mg	ESI Pharma
	5 mg	
	10 mg	
Micronor (norethindrone)	0.35 mg	Ortho
Provera (MPA*)	2.5 mg	Upjohn
	5 mg	
	10 mg	

* Medroxyprogesterone acetate

the case, then estrogen may be given alone. Women using estrogen alone require periodic testing to monitor the growth of the lining of the uterus.

In individuals without a uterus, oral estrogen or the transdermal patch can be administered for 25 days each calendar month, since there is no danger of buildup of the lining of the uterus.

Cyclic Combined

Estrogen and progestin are taken the first 3 weeks of each month and nothing is taken the remainder of the month; vaginal withdrawal bleeding will usually occur.

Cyclic Estrogen And Cyclic Progestin

Estrogens are given for the first 21 days of each calendar month and progestins are usually added during the last 1 to 2 weeks of the estrogen schedule. After the 21st of the month, no medication is given and vaginal withdrawal bleeding usually results. The most common oral progestins given are medroxyprogesterone acetate (MPA) at 5 or 10 mg per day or norethindrone acetate at 2.5 mg or 5 mg.

Continuous Unopposed Estrogen

As stated earlier, this treatment is not recommended for individuals with an intact uterus because of the danger of uterine cancer, but may be used with individuals who do not have a uterus. Estrogen is taken daily in the form of a tablet, or the patch is worn continuously and changed periodically according to manufacturer's recommendations. A continuous program has several advantages including a resemblance of the more normal pattern of estrogen production by the ovary and better adherence because it is easier to remember to take a pill daily or apply the transdermal patch than to adjust schedules.

Continuous Estrogen And Cyclic Progestin

Estrogen is taken continuously orally or the transdermal patch is worn daily. The progestin is usually added during the first one to two weeks each month. Vaginal bleeding may occur. One advantage of this method is that it is easy for many people.

Continuous Combined Estrogen/Progestin Regimen

One of the most frequent complaints of women on any of the combined estrogen and progestin treatment regimes is the withdrawal bleeding that occurs, as well as the premenstrual discomforts associated with the administration of cyclic progestin. An alternate method, which reduces the likelihood of significant bleeding while still offering the protective effect of a progestin, is combined treatment which is taken continuously. Oral estrogen is taken daily, or transdermal patches are worn continuously and the progestin dose is decreased since it is given daily. There are no pill or patch-free days. Although many women experience irregular episodes of bleeding during the first few months, most women will be free of bleeding episodes after approximately six months of continuous therapy. In general, advantages include convenience and discontinuation of withdrawal bleeding after four to six months while maintaining protection for the uterus, osteoporosis protection, and favorable impact on blood lipids.

Progestins Only

The use of progestins alone to control menopausal symptoms is another area of controversy. This therapy does seem to offer relief for hot flashes. If indeed more studies do support the previous information we have on the benefits of progestin on bone, then there is some merit to the use of progestin. Yet, control of the other menopausal problems involving the urinary tract, vagina, and cardiovascular system must be considered. Even disqualifying the negative effects on blood lipids, what are the benefits of using progestins alone? To date, there seems to be little information that tells us that progestins will protect the postmenopausal female from heart disease. The same is true of progestins and breast cancer. If it is true that progestins do offer protection against breast cancer, what happens to the heart?

This treatment regimen alone points out the decisions women are faced with regarding treatment programs. Women are faced with increasingly difficult choices. Should women be faced with asking, "Do I want to die from breast cancer, heart disease, or complications of osteoporosis?" Perhaps it is better to choose a drug that has at least been around for a long time and has been studied extensively, even if some of the studies are less than perfect. A great deal of information is out there that has found that estrogen helps keep bones and hearts healthy.

WHO NEEDS ESTROGEN THERAPY?

Interestingly enough not all postmenopausal women need estrogen replacement, since some produce sufficient estrogen

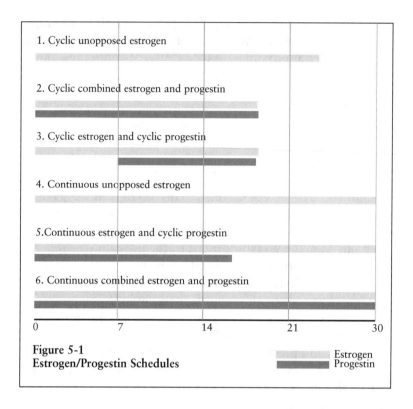

Figure 5-1
Estrogen/Progestin Schedules

Estrogen
Progestin

which prevents many of the symptoms associated with menopause as well as osteoporosis and cardiovascular changes normally associated with decreased estrogen levels. It has been suggested these women receive progestin periodically, every three
to six months to determine estrogen status and to start shedding of the uterine lining to prevent the risk of uterine cancer.[5]

SIDE EFFECTS OF ESTROGENS AND PROGESTINS

Although there are women who should not take HRT for a
variety of reasons which will be discussed later, there are some
side effects of which anyone choosing to take HRT should be
aware. Not all women experience these side effects, and even

those who do usually experience them to a limited degree. Some of the side effects are

- nausea (the most common side effect), short term
- fluid retention
- increase in severity of migraine headaches (may be related to fluid retention)
- yellowing of the skin and/or the eyes (rare)
- a spotty discoloration of the skin or skin rashes (rare)
- breast tenderness or enlargement, short term
- irregular bleeding or spotting, short term
- enlargement of benign (nonmalignant) fibroids in the uterus
- vaginal yeast infections (rare)
- excessive vaginal secretions (usually associated with high doses of estrogen)
- mental depression
- hair loss or abnormal hairiness
- increase or decrease in weight, and
- changes in sex drive

Many times an adjustment in the dose of estrogen may eliminate or control some of these side effects. For some of the premenstrual syndrome (PMS) side effects such as breast tenderness, bloating, irritability, and depression, adjusting the dose, using another form of progestin, or adding a low-dose diuretic during the last few days of the progestin treatment period will eliminate these problems.

One of the concerns with the use of progestins has been their negative effect on blood lipids or cholesterol levels which affect the heart. Some studies have shown that progestins counteract the good effects of estrogens on the lipids (estrogens raise the high density lipids and lower the low density lipids and progestins do just the opposite). What some studies have shown is, that if adequate doses of estrogen are used, progestin does not cancel these good effects by acting on HDL (High Density Lipoproteins). What is not known is whether progestin works against estrogen's good effects on other parts of the cardiovascular system, such as blood flow, blood components, and blood vessel tone.

Recent results of a 3 year study, the "Postmenopausal estrogen/progestin interventions (PEPI) Trial," one of the few random, formally controlled studies, have shown that estrogen in combination with progestin does reduce cardiovascular risk. This study "debunked" many of the uncertainties and even some myths that have surrounded HRT. The study did have some limitations because various types of progestins and estrogens were not tested. Nevertheless this study is not without merit and the results warrant a review:

- Estrogen did not lose its beneficial lipid effect on the cardiovascular system when combined with progesterone. HDL "good" cholesterol was increased in all study groups. Women who took natural progesterone which is not generally available in the U.S. showed an increase in HDL. Users of unopposed estrogen or estrogen alone had the highest HDL levels. The increase in HDL was not as great for women who took the progestins, the synthetic form of progesterone, although their HDL levels were still significantly higher than those women who received placebos.

- HRT did not increase blood pressure as was previously believed.

- HRT did not increase blood clotting factors; it decreased them.

- Probably one of the most controversial issues surrounding HRT was that the cardiovascular benefits were due to the "healthy user" syndrome, e.g., the healthy user visits the doctor more frequently, is more likely to engage in exercise, and watches her diet. Healthy women in the test population would show strong cardiovascular results because of their already healthy condition. Yet the women who received no treatment (some who were also healthy women) did not have the same positive cardiovascular effects as those who received HRT.

The PEPI study further confirmed that adding a progestin to the estrogen treatment regime provided a good overall effect. An increase in the uterine lining of those women who were on estrogen only makes combination hormone therapy prudent if not mandatory for women with a uterus. The addition of a progestin alleviates the excessive growth of the lining of the uterus and preserves the estrogen's favorable effect on the cardiovascular system. Probably of greatest importance will be whether these factors over time will result in less cardiovascular disease; observational studies suggest it will.[7,8] "Thus, for women whose primary concern is heart disease, HRT is continuing to look better and better."[9]

CONTRAINDICATIONS

In the past, many of the reasons for not using estrogen in certain individuals were based on the complications of high-dose contraceptives. Current information indicates that more women than previously thought can take estrogen including those with a wide range of medical problems. Current reasons not to take estrogen include:

- vaginal bleeding when the cause is unknown
- active liver disease
- active clotting disorders
- known or suspected pregnancy
- known or suspected estrogen-dependent tumors, and
- known or suspected past or recent history of breast cancer (although there have been some recent changes in this thinking which will be discussed later in this chapter)

EVEN PROBLEM CASES DESERVE ESTROGEN

Even for some women with contraindications, estrogen may be prescribed. For example, if a harmless cause for vaginal bleeding is found and liver and clotting disorders are successfully treated, then some authorities believe that estrogen can be given. Transdermal methods seem to be especially useful for individuals with clotting problems, past liver disease, and gallbladder disease since this transdermal method bypasses the liver and prevents the liver's effect on clotting factors.[10,11]

Estrogen may have mixed results for women with endometriosis, fibrocystic breast disease, and migraine headaches. Depending upon the severity of the problem, a trial period of HRT may be in order; but if problems become more severe as a result of the therapy, an alteration of the program is necessary. If other medications alleviate symptoms, the dosage level does not have to change; but if they do not, a reduction or discontinuation of the medication is required.[11] Other situations which one might wonder about include:

- Individuals with a prior history of ovarian or cervical cancer can use ERT (Estrogen replacement therapy).

- The presence of cardiovascular disease, diabetes, or high blood pressure does not prevent the use of estrogen therapy. As a matter of fact, those individuals with heart disease on ERT show a higher survival rate than those not receiving ERT. Death due to stroke also appears to be reduced with ERT.

- Gall bladder disease should no longer be a contraindication to ERT, although the establishment of a real cause-and-effect relationship has not been discovered. According to some experts, the benefits and risks of estrogen therapy outweigh the risks encountered with existing gall bladder disease.[11]

Decisions About Risks

As discussed earlier, with any drug, there is a benefit/risk decision. Taking aspirin is not without some risk. Taking an antibiotic for an infection is not without risk. The choice must be based on what selection is going to provide the greatest benefit. Hormone replacement therapy has important benefits but also some risks. Whether the risks of estrogen use are acceptable because of the benefits is a decision that must be made by you in consultation with your health professional.

Once you decide to take HRT, you can reduce some of the risks or side effects by carefully watching your treatment and bringing anything that seems out of the ordinary to the attention of your health care provider. See your health care provider regularly and follow his/her recommendations carefully. Do not hesitate to ask questions.

CANCER OF THE UTERUS

The relationship of hormones to cancer of the uterus has long been recognized. Uterine cancer risk is decreased when menopause occurs at an earlier age, when oral contraceptives have been used, and with a greater number of pregnancies, whereas increased body weight in both premenopausal and postmenopausal women and use of estrogen replacement therapy increase the risk.

An association between the increasing incidence of uterine cancer and estrogens was made in 1975 when it was reported that the risk of uterine cancer was greater among women using estrogen (alone or "unopposed") as opposed to those who had never used it. Since then numerous studies have confirmed this association. The risk of developing cancer of the uterus increases the longer the usage and the higher the dose. Some studies have shown that the cancer risk stayed high for 8 to more than 15 years after stopping estrogen treatment. Others have found the risk of uterine cancer associated with unopposed estrogen therapy to be lower than that previously reported. These decreased risks appear to be dose dependent, meaning the lower the dose, the lower the risk or incidence. Suggestions have also been made that the cancers associated with estrogen use are of an earlier stage and a lower severity compared with those that arise in estrogen nonusers.[12]

During the late 1970s, the value of adding progestin to the estrogen therapy treatment plan was clear. By 1981 the addition of progestin to estrogen therapy had been shown to reduce uterine lining abnormalities. The use of this combined

157

hormone replacement therapy by postmenopausal women has increased steadily since then.

While estrogen causes the uterine lining to thicken, progestin works by either decreasing the growth of this lining or to causing the lining to shed. How the progestin is taken will determine which effect will occur. Taking estrogen and progestin on a continuous basis will cause a decreased growth of the uterine lining. The shedding process happens when the progestin is taken on a cyclic schedule which causes the uterine lining to shed on a cyclic basis also. When following a cyclic schedule, progestin is taken for at least 12 to 14 days.

Women who take progestin with estrogen have been found to have no increased risk of developing uterine cancer when compared to postmenopausal women who do not take estrogen. In fact, the addition of progestin to ERT during the late 1970s has shifted the national incidence of uterine cancer. However, it must be understood that no progestin will prevent all uterine cancers since there are some cancers that are not hormone related. And finally, according to most experts, no rationale exists for giving progestin to women who have had a hysterectomy.

BREAST CANCER AND HORMONES

Estimates show that 1 woman in 8 will have breast cancer during her lifetime and about 1 in 33 will die from breast cancer. According to the American Cancer Society, breast cancer incidence rates for women have increased about 2% per year since 1980, but recently have leveled off. Some of the recent rise in rates is believed to be due to a marked increase in mammography utilization, allowing the detection of early stage breast cancer, frequently before it is apparent physically. Despite the continuing rise in the incidence of breast cancer, the death rate has remained fairly stable over the past 50 years which seems to be largely due to earlier detection. Other reasons for a longer-term increase in breast cancer are not yet understood.[13] Furthermore, the information currently available suggests that the death rate is falling in White women, but not in Blacks, perhaps because of early detection and improved treatment.

Breast cancer risk rises with aging, yet the small percentage of women currently using HRT cannot justify the magnitude of this risk. Nevertheless, since three-quarters of all breast cancer cannot yet be attributed to any known specific causes, all women should be treated as being at risk, to some degree, for breast cancer.[13]

Risk Factors

If all women are considered to be at risk, then all women should be aware of the risk factors associated with breast cancer. These include:

- age, over 50
- personal or family history of breast cancer
- menstrual periods at an early age
- menopause at a late age
- postmenopausal ERT (questionable)
- never having children
- having first child after age 30
- higher education and socioeconomic status
- obesity
- high fat diet (questionable)

Possible Signs And Symptoms

A wise woman will learn the possible signs and symptoms of breast cancer.

Breast Changes To Note Are
- lump or thickening
- swelling
- dimpling
- skin irritation or scaling

- distortion or retraction
- pain
- nipple tenderness or discharge

A health care professional should be consulted if any of these signs and symptoms are present.[13]

HRT And My Breast, Am I Safe?

Again, studies give conflicting information on the relationship of HRT to breast cancer. But, the news is not really bad! Decades of research have failed to definitely prove that HRT absolutely causes breast cancer. Higher rates that are apparent in European studies are supposedly due to the kind of hormones used (many of which are synthetic estrogens), higher doses, and characteristics of the women who receive them. Furthermore, a variety of androgens and progestins (which may differ from those used in this country) have been used more frequently in Europe.

In the United States, at least 70 percent of the estrogen product sold is Premarin (Wyeth-Ayerst Laboratories). The use of progestins in the United States has been in existence for almost two decades, and the one most frequently used is Provera [(MPA) Upjohn]. Therefore, many of the studies include the use of Premarin or Premarin and Provera. A final evaluation of all of these studies has shown either a modest to small increased risk to no increased risk.[14,15] However, the most recent information coming from the Nurses' Health Study which started in 1976, tells us that the longer the use of estrogen, especially in older women, the greater the risk for breast cancer.[16]

To complicate matters even more, other studies are telling us that estrogen therapy need not be avoided in individuals with a history of breast cancer. An article published in *Menopause: The Journal of the North American Menopause Society* reported that in one large scale study there were fewer recurrences and no deaths in estrogen-progestin users with a history of breast cancer as compared with another group of patients with a history of breast cancer who took no hormones.[17]

For those who do choose HRT with some degree of apprehension regarding breast cancer, certain actions can provide some degree of reasonable security. Yearly mammograms, monthly breast self-examination, and an annual breast examination by a health care provider for early detection of breast cancer will virtually eliminate the possibility of developing undetected breast cancer.

Mammography A mammogram is vital to early detection of breast cancer and is a safe, low-dose x-ray picture of the breast which can often show breast changes like lumps long before they can be felt. And the sooner breast cancer is detected and treated, the greater the chances for a cure. Mammography, either in combination with clinical breast examination or alone, has been known to reduce breast cancer mortality, particularly in older women.

The Department of Health and Human Services Agency for Health Care Policy and Research recommends seven steps to breast health.[18]

1. Get regular exams.
- Get a breast exam from your health professional when you get your physical exam, every 3 years for women 20 to 40 and every year for those over 40.[13]
- Get a mammogram as often as your health professional recommends. Ask your health professional when to schedule your next mammogram.
  - The American Cancer Society recommends that women who have no signs or symptoms should have a mammogram by age 40
    - women ages 40 to 49 should have a mammogram every 1 to 2 years
    - women age 50 and over should have a mammogram every year
- Check your breasts each month. Again, the American Cancer society recommends a monthly breast self-examination for women 20 years and older. Your health professional can show you how or you may refer to Figure

5-2 for the appropriate way to do your self-examination. These three exams, the self-examination, examination by a health professional and mammogram, can help you and your health professional learn what is normal for your breasts and what may be a sign of problems.

2. Choose a quality facility

- Your health professional may refer you to a mammography facility, or you may select one that is most convenient for you

- A new law, called the Mammography Quality Standards Act, requires all mammography facilities except those of a Veterans Health Administration (VHA) facility to be certified by the Food and Drug Administration (FDA) effective October 1, 1994. To be certified, facilities must meet standards for the equipment they use, the people who work there, and the records they keep. VHA has its own high-quality mammography program, similar to the FDA's program.

- Make certain the mammography facility you choose is certified by the FDA unless it is a VHA facility. A certified mammography facility should have a certificate on display in a place where it may be easily seen and read.

- To find a certified facility, ask your health professional or call the National Cancer Institute Cancer Information Service at 1-800-4-CANCER.

3. Schedule the mammogram when your breasts should be least tender.

- For those women who are premenopausal, the best time for a mammogram may be about a week-and-a-half after your period. For the postmenopausal woman the best time will depend on whether you are on HRT and whether your breasts are sensitive at certain times of the month. If you are not on HRT, this may not be a problem.

4. Give and get important information when you schedule the mammogram.

- The mammography facility may ask you questions over the telephone or when you have your mammogram. The requested information may include:

- name, address, phone number
- age
- name, address, phone number of any facility where you may have had a previous mammogram
- any breast disease in your family
- any current problems with your breasts
- past problems with your breasts, breast biopsies, or breast surgeries
- whether you have breast implants
- name, address, phone number of your health professional
- other personal information such as
  - whether you are pregnant or nursing
  - the timing of your menstrual period or when menopause began
  - anything that might make it more difficult to do a mammogram such as large breasts

5. Know what to expect.

- When you have a mammogram, you stand in front of a special x-ray machine. Each breast is placed on a platform that holds the x-ray film.
- The breast is then gradually pressed against the platform by a specially designed clear plastic plate. Some pressure is needed for a few seconds to make sure the x-rays show as much of the breast as possible.
- This pressure is not harmful to your breast. In fact, flattening the breast lowers the x-ray dose needed.
- Studies show that most women do not find a mammogram painful for the short time needed to take the picture. Try to relax.

6. Come prepared.

- Wear a two-piece outfit as you will have to remove only your top

- Do not use deodorant, talcum powder, or lotion under your arms or near the breasts that day. These products can show up on the x-ray picture.

- Ask the facilities where you had mammograms before to release the films to you and bring them with you if possible. Your new mammogram can be compared with the earlier ones to see if there have been any changes.

7. Follow up on your results.

- More than likely your mammogram will be normal, BUT DO NOT ASSUME that your mammogram is normal just because you have not received the results. If you have not received your screening results within 10 days, call your doctor or the mammography facility.

- If your screening mammogram shows anything unusual, talk to your health professional as soon as possible about what you should do next. Your health professional may schedule another kind of mammogram known as a diagnostic mammogram or recommend a biopsy which is a small piece of breast tissue obtained for study under a microscope.

- Whenever a mammogram uncovers a problem or a need to check something further

  - make sure you understand what you need to do next

  - always get results of any test that you have had

  - ask questions about your results if you do not understand something

- If you do not have a health care professional, you will need to find one if you have an abnormal mammogram. Ask the mammography facility to help you find a health care professional, then make an appointment right away so you can discuss your results and what should be done next.

- Mammography is very effective, but it does not detect all breast problems. If you have a breast lump or change at any time, even if your last mammogram was normal, see a health professional as soon as possible.

REMEMBER YOU ARE IN CHARGE OF YOUR BREAST HEALTH!

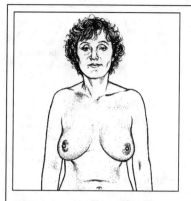

STEP 1. Stand in front of a mirror that is large enough for you to see your breasts clearly. Check each breast for anything unusual. Check the skin for puckering, dimpling, or scaliness. Look for a discharge from the nipples.

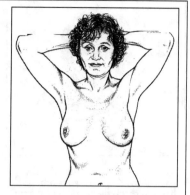

Do steps 2 and 3 to check for any change in the shape or contour of your breasts. As you do these steps, you should feel your chest muscles tighten.

STEP 2. Watching closely in the mirror, clasp your hands behind your head and press your hands forward.

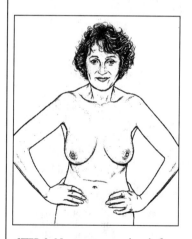

STEP 3. Next press your hands firmly on your hips and bend slightly toward the mirror as you pull your shoulders and elbows forward.

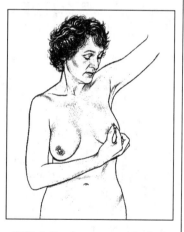

STEP 4. Gently squeeze each nipple and look for discharge.

Figure 5-2. Breast self-examination

(continued)

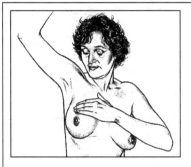

breast in a circle. Move around the breast in smaller and smaller circles, gradually working toward the nipple. Don't forget to check the underarm and upper chest areas, too.

STEP 5.   Raise one arm. Use the pads of the fingers of your other hand to check the breast and the surrounding area—firmly, carefully, thoroughly. Some women like to use lotion or powder to help their fingers glide easily over the skin. The shower is also a good place to conduct this part of the examination since fingers will glide easily over soapy skin, and then you can concentrate on feeling for changes. Feel for any unusual lump or mass under the skin.

Feel the tissue by pressing your fingers in small, overlapping areas about the size of a dime. To be sure you cover your whole breast, take your time and follow a definite pattern: lines, circles, wedges. The important thing is to cover the whole breast and to pay special attention to the area between the breast and the underarm, including the underarm itself. Check the area above the breast, up to the collarbone and all the way over to your shoulder.

LINES: Start in the underarm area and move your fingers downward little by little until they are below the breast. Then move your fingers slightly toward the middle and slowly move back up. Go up and down until you cover the whole area.

CIRCLES: Beginning at the outer edge of your breast, move your fingers slowly around the whole

WEDGES: Starting at the outer edge of the breast, move your fingers toward the nipple and back to the edge. Check your whole breast, covering one small wedge-shaped section at a time. Be sure to check the underarm area and the upper chest.

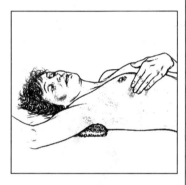

STEP 6. It is important to repeat step 5 while you are lying down. Lie flat on your back, with one arm over your head and a pillow or folded towel under the shoulder. This position flattens the breast and makes it easier to check. Check each breast and the area around it very carefully using one of the patterns described above.

*Remember, BSE is not a substitute for routine mammograms or regular breast exams by a health professional.

Source: U.S. Department Of Health And Human Services. National Cancer Institute. National Institutes of Health Publication No. 94-1556. Bethesda, Maryland 20892. Revised July 1993.

FIBROCYSTIC CONDITION

Actually this term is another name for chronic cystic mastitis and describes a number of conditions found in the breast. Some may consider this a premalignant disorder, but most incidents of fibrocystic changes do not lead to breast cancer.

The actual cause of fibrocystic changes is unknown but it is believed to be an exaggerated response of breast tissue to the ebb and flow of ovarian hormones, mainly estrogen and progesterone. Most women who have discomfort from fibrocystic changes may have some relief after menopause, yet the discomfort may reoccur with estrogen replacement therapy. Caffeine and nicotine are believed to be contributors although this is not an absolute. Discontinuing either or both is harmless and may help with relieving fibrocystic symptoms. Vitamin E and vitamin A are reported to be helpful, but data about these vitamins are not conclusive and too much of either is not good. Further research is needed in this area. Continuous surveillance with regular breast examinations and mammograms is the best preventive measure since a definite relationship between fibrocystic changes and breast cancer has not been established.

MENOPAUSE AND BEYOND WITHOUT HRT: WHAT ARE THE CHOICES?

For those women who either cannot or choose not to take HRT life is not just "gloom and doom." Exercise, diet, and lifestyle changes have been shown to be viable alternatives in the treatment of many of the symptoms and problems associated with the postmenopausal period of a woman's life. Early changes in one's diet and lifestyle in addition to aerobic, weight-bearing, and muscle-strengthening exercises are proven to be beneficial no matter what "ails" you. The bothersome menopausal hot flashes, mood changes, depression, fatigue, and insomnia as described earlier can many times be alleviated or at least controlled with the use of diet, exercise, and changes in lifestyle, not to mention improvement in the more problematic areas of heart and bone health. To maximize these effects, it has already been stated that estrogen is required; but for those who cannot or choose not to use HRT opportunities are always available that will contribute to one's well being as well as contribute to one's overall health. These nondrug alternatives are described within the respective sections with further detailed information in Chapter 6 on exercise and diet.

Treatment Alternatives

Herbal medicine, vitamins, homeopathy, and acupressure have all been proposed as viable alternatives to HRT. To date, there is very little or no scientific information to acknowledge and support most of these treatments. Most of the success of these remedies is based upon hearsay, but much is still being written about these alternative remedies or treatment programs in magazines and books. Health stores and even some pharmacies are becoming the "shopping malls" for these products. All of them claim to be the real or natural way to combat the woes of menopause. Women are trying all of these remedies based on information from friends, magazines, individuals selling the products, and even some health professionals. Are they harmless? Some perhaps are. Some have estrogenic properties and behave in the body just as prescribed estrogens; but the dose is difficult to determine because of the erratic amounts contained in these herbs. For example ginseng is an herbal source of estrogen and therefore a form of hormone therapy. It can be effective in treating hot flashes as well as other symptoms of menopause, but carries the same risks as estrogen replacement therapy.[19] It is also a stimulant and taking too much may cause insomnia and anxiety.[20] Likewise, the use of the herb dong quai is an estrogen precursor and those individuals who should not be taking estrogen should not be taking this herb. Estrogen in any form has the potential for stimulating growth of the uterine lining in women with a uterus. Thus these women need periodic biopsies of the uterine lining or require a progestin.

Herbal therapy may indeed be a useful alternative to hormonal therapy; the problem is that there has not been enough research to evaluate its safety and effectiveness. Until more studies are available, caution should be exercised in the use of any herbs. Before embarking on your own treatment program it is always best to seek the advice of your health professional. .

Dietary Or Phyto-estrogen   Dietary or phyto-estrogen is a general term used to define compounds that have weak estrogenic activity. Flaxseed and soybean are particularly abundant sources of these kinds of estrogens. Flaxseed is not a commonly consumed food product, but soy protein is. Soy protein makes up a significant part of the traditional Japanese diet, In Japan, hot flashes in menopausal women are relatively uncommon in those who consume the traditional diet. For this reason, some believe that these food products can be used safely in postmenopausal women in place of estrogen replacement therapy; because it is a food product, many believe it is therefore safer. The problem again is the danger for those who should not be taking estrogen, and for those women with a uterus, where the excessive growth of the uterine lining could lead to a precancerous state. Although soy protein may some day prove to be an alternative nondrug approach, the potential for its use in the postmenopausal period remains to be investigated.[21,22]

Yams   Likewise yams, both wild and domestic, have been suggested to play a role as a substitute for estrogen replacement. Domestic yams are more easily accessible and need to be eaten raw and in large quantities. These yams contain very small amounts of estrogenic compounds which are inactivated by cooking, and vary from yam to yam and crop to crop. Years ago yams were used to manufacture estrogen for human and animal use; today, the urine from pregnant mares is more readily available and more widely used. Yams also contain diosgenin which can also be used in the manufacture of progesterone.[23]

Wild mexican yams contain a substance similar to progesterone which relieve hot flashes. These yams are available in the form of pills, suppositories, and cream. Controlling dosages of skin cream, in particular is very difficult, and excessive amounts can cause fluid retention, irritability, and weight gain just as the synthetic forms.[20]

Still, there are those who claim that "estrogen is the wrong hormonal treatment for most post-menopausal women and natural progesterone, derived from wild yams and applied to the skin, is much more effective against osteoporosis and has no side effects".[24] One may ask, who is correct and which advice should I follow? For the most part, the scientific literature to date has not advocated the use of a treatment protocol such as this. Certainly, one of the major drawbacks to an application of this kind is controlling the dose of progesterone.

Vitamin E   Vitamins have also been suggested as possible alternatives to control hot flashes. Vitamin E is one of those vitamins which was tested in the 1940s and 1950s with mixed results because of the way the studies were conducted. The primary purpose of vitamin E is to preserve the health of body tissues. Vitamin E deficiency is rare except in premature infants and in individuals who cannot absorb fat normally. No strong evidence exists that large doses of vitamin E are harmful. The recommended dose of vitamin E is 400 to 800 IU and megadoses of up to 50 times the recommended dose can elevate blood lipids, interfere with the normal clotting mechanism in the blood and impair white blood cell activity (white blood cells fight infection). Muscle weakness and fatigue have also been found in doses that exceed 1000 units a day.[25]

Increasing foods rich in vitamin E may be a more sensible approach than taking high doses of vitamin E. Vitamin E is widely distributed in foods such as wheat germ, spinach, whole grains, legumes, nuts, dark green leafy vegetables, soybean products, and vegetable oils (corn, soy, sunflower, safflower, cottonseed).

Homeopathy   Homeopathy has been proposed as another

alternative and is a method of treating diseases with very small doses of a drug, which if given in very large doses in a healthy person would produce symptoms similar to the disease itself. For example, sepia is used to treat a dry vagina; lycopodium, a poor memory; and pulsatilla, insomnia.

Acupuncture   Even acupuncture, new to this country but long used in China, Japan, and other countries, has been used to treat menopausal problems either alone or in combination with herbs and other remedies. Controversy regarding pressure points and needling techniques does exist. Although acupuncture use for pain control is well known and has been studied, the use of acupuncture in the treatment of menopausal symptoms is less known.

Deciding   There is no doubt that some of these alternatives may have merit, but how can one make these determinations? Beware of the claims that are made. Until adequate and reliable research is conducted, caution regarding the safety of these different methods should be exercised. Furthermore, if you are apprehensive regarding the claims made about hormone replacement therapy which have actually been examined for many years, then you ought to be equally cautious about the use of these remedies. In other words, apply the same prudent standards for both. Discuss them with your health care provider.

Use of these remedies requires extensive research to determine the safety and effectiveness of these methods, not only to protect the women who use them, but also to prevent women from wasting their time and money on methods that are unlikely to yield positive results.[25,26]

BENEFITS AND CONCERNS

Estrogen replacement therapy offers significant benefits to nearly all postmenopausal women, especially those for whom the menopause occurred at an early age. Symptoms of decreased estrogen levels such as hot flashes, night sweats with

subsequent sleep disturbances, vaginal dryness, painful intercourse, and urinary disturbances will obviously improve when
estrogen is given. Women at high risk for cardiovascular disease or who already have cardiovascular disease may particularly benefit from estrogen use. The increased risk for endometrial and breast cancer with estrogen replacement therapy is
low in comparison with its protective effect against cardiovascular disease. The effects of estrogen on bone and the prevention of osteoporosis have been well documented. Experts in
the field of osteoporosis acknowledge that estrogen replacement is the single most important factor in combating this disease. Conversely, women with absolute contraindications to
estrogen treatment, such as those with active breast cancer,
acute liver disease, or estrogen-related blood clots, should not
receive estrogen regardless of the severity of the symptoms.

Benefits

In summary, the two most important benefits of estrogen
replacement therapy are the reduction in both osteoporosis
and heart disease.

Prevention Of Osteoporosis   As stated earlier, one million
women suffer fractures due to osteoporosis annually and several others have the disease and do not know it. The costs
both in terms of money and loss of life or inability to participate in the usual activities of daily living are staggering.
Research has shown that estrogen prevents a decline in bone
mass especially when combined with exercise and an adequate calcium intake.

Prevention Of Cardiovascular Disease   Cardiovascular disease which is relatively nonexistent prior to the postmenopausal years is the major cause of death in older women,
accounting for ten times the number of deaths caused by
breast cancer. There is a vast amount of evidence that says
estrogen replacement decreases the risk of death and also the
incidence of heart disease in women. High blood pressure also
seems to be less common in those on ERT, as is stroke.

Concerns

Cancer Of The Uterus   The increased risk for cancer of the uterus, formerly a big concern with ERT, has virtually been eliminated with the use of progestin.

Blood Lipids   The negative effects, of progestins on blood lipids, have not been shown with lower progestin doses. Furthermore adjusting both the estrogen and progestin doses seem to alleviate this problem.

Breast Health   The more than 50 studies conducted in the last 20 years on the effects of estrogen on the breast have not shown us there is an absolute relationship between estrogen use and breast cancer, although there may be a small increase in long time users.

Bloating And Irritability   The uncomfortable side effects of bloating and irritability sometimes associated with progestins can be modified with the use of different progestins and adjustment of the dose.

Monthly Bleeding   Monthly bleeding can be eliminated with the use of continuous administration of both estrogen and progestin or alternate schedules such as progestin every 3 months or even less. Some of these newer methods require more frequent visits to your health professional to make certain the lining of the uterus is not becoming too thick.

Knowledge Is The Key   Although it seems most of the recent evidence is reassuring, and regular examinations by your health care provider in addition to your own surveillance should prevent any possible problems, there are no absolutes. At this point, you should have a good understanding of the risks and benefits which will enable you, in consultation with your health care provider, to make the choice that is best for you. The extensive reference list, located in the back of the book, includes some of the best scientific literature available. You don't need to have a medical library nearby to obtain any of these articles. Your local community library can request them through the interlibrary loan system, and all you have to do is provide them with the information given on each article listed in the Reference List. All of this will further assist you in your decision making.[27]

AND NOW FOR THE FINAL QUESTION: WHEN IS IT SAFE TO STOP?

Many women are unaware that they may still be fertile once menstrual periods become irregular. Although the average age of menopause is 51, nearly 30% of women ages 50 to 54 remain fertile.[28] Since menopause is not officially defined until a year has passed without a menstrual period, the time in between can be crucial. To be sure pregnancy does not occur during this time frame, contraception or natural family planning practice should be continued until menstruation is absent for one year. FSH/LH (follicle stimulating hormone/luteinizing hormone) testing can determine menopausal status for those women who continue on oral contraceptives.

Some authorities recommend the use of oral contraceptives to approximately age 50 with a transition at that time to hormone replacement therapy. Thus, women may find themselves taking oral contraceptives to prevent pregnancy and then taking hormone replacement therapy after menopause for the remainder of their lives. For example, a sexually active woman between the ages of 42 and 55 with hot flashes, no periods for the last 6 months, and FSH levels of more than 40 mIU/mL is probably ready for HRT; whereas, a woman in the same age bracket with regular or irregular periods and FSH levels of less that 40 mIU/mL should probably continue with oral contraceptives or other means of contraception to avoid pregnancy.

The next question "when is it safe to stop" in terms of prevention of osteoporosis and cardiovascular disease presents another big question mark. By now you are aware of the convincing evidence of estrogen on preservation of both bone and heart health. You have read that many experts are recommending long term use of estrogen for both osteoporosis and cardiovascular disease prevention, even into the 70s and 80s, since risk increases with age. Is this good or bad? There is no definite answer. The unknown is the lack of information on long-term use of estrogen. However, by now you have a vast body of knowledge to draw upon, and resources that have been provided in this book, which will enable you to make the best decision possible. A variety of treatment methods and a wealth of information are available to help you maintain a healthy and productive lifestyle.

In summary, no decision is final! Each woman should review any decision she has made on an annual basis with her health care provider. Our bodies change and so does the information available to us, thus the pros and cons of new information must be evaluated. Of equal importance is keeping your health care provider up-to-date on how you are managing your life. Don't attempt to "do it alone." Let them be your "best friend and colleague" on your road to good health.

Chapter Six

HOW TO LEAD A
HEALTHY LIFE

F
ew of us need to be told that a nutritious diet, adequate
sleep, a manageable stress-free life, and vigorous exercise could probably lead to a healthier existence. But
couple the seemingly incredible will power and luck needed
to create such a life with the devastating concept that the perfect female must have a tiny size 6 to size 10 figure, flawless
skin, and manageable hair and the goal becomes unattainable. Every plan must begin with realistic expectations. A
health plan begins with an acceptance of who you are and the
willingness to explore who you can be. Artificial convention,
or a model of the "perfect woman" plays no part here.
Recognizing the difference between realistic and unattainable
goals is the first step in creating a health plan; realizing that
we have the power to make our goals happen is the second.

Much useful information has been explored in the preceding chapters, but the trick is how to pull it all together. Do not
worry! In an age where new information surfaces daily, some
basic guidelines have survived and serve as an anchor for
shaping our health plans. This chapter will include discussions
on dietary guidelines first and exercise guidelines last.

WOMEN AND NUTRITION

The "Dietary Guidelines for Americans" developed by the
Departments of Health and Human Services (DHHS) and
Agriculture (USDA) are the best, most up-to-date advice from

nutrition scientists and are the basis of federal nutrition policy. These guidelines are not for children under the age of 2 or for infants, neither are they for persons with certain types of medical problems. Following the Guidelines can reduce the chance of getting certain diseases and lead to better health.[1,2] The Dietary Guidelines are:

- eat a variety of foods
- maintain a healthy weight
- choose a diet with minimal total fat, saturated fat, and cholesterol
- choose a diet with plenty of vegetables, fruits, and grain products
- use sugar and salt/sodium only in moderation
- if you drink alcoholic beverages, do so in moderation

Let us explore each idea.

Eat A Variety Of Foods

To meet the requirement to "eat a variety of foods" you need more than 40 different nutrients to maintain good health. No single food can supply all the needed nutrients in the correct amounts, so a variety of foods are recommended, not just a few highly fortified foods or supplements. For example, milk supplies calcium but little iron; meat supplies iron but little calcium. One way to assure variety—and with it, an enjoyable and nutritious diet—is to choose food each day from five major food groups.

The Food Guide Pyramid The U.S. Department of Agriculture (USDA) and the Department of Health and Human Services (DHHS) have developed The Food Guide Pyramid, which aids in choosing the selection and amounts of food from each food group to get the nutrients needed each day. These Guidelines are designed to monitor the intake of calories, fat, saturated fat, cholesterol, sugar, sodium, and alcohol. The Pyramid focuses on fat, curbing the intake of total and saturated fat, because most Americans' diets are too high in fat.

The Pyramid is an outline of what should be eaten each day, not a rigid prescription. A general guide, it allows for a healthful diet to meet each individual's needs. Before reviewing the Food Guide Pyramid, two simple concepts must be explained. Each of the five groups provide some, but not all of the needed nutrients, and foods in one group cannot replace those in another. No one group is more important than another; all are necessary. The Pyramid visually demonstrates the proportion of intake necessary for a healthy diet. Fats should constitute the smallest portion of a daily menu, while foods in the bread group should constitute the largest portion.

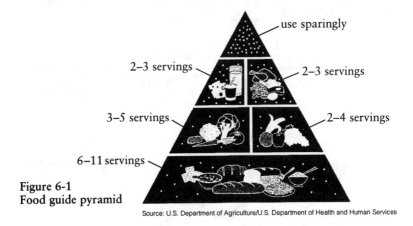

use sparingly

2–3 servings

2–3 servings

3–5 servings

2–4 servings

6–11 servings

Figure 6-1
Food guide pyramid

Source: U.S. Department of Agriculture/U.S. Department of Health and Human Services

- The small tip of the Pyramid shows fats oils, and sweets. Foods in this category include salad dressings and oils, cream, butter, margarine, sugars, soft drinks, candies, and sweet desserts. These foods provide calories and little else nutritionally. Calories that provide little to no nutritional value are called empty calories. Use them sparingly.

- The next level contains two separate groups of foods. Both groups have a predominantly animal source. The dairy group includes milk, yogurt, and cheese. The meat group includes meats, poultry, fish, dry beans, eggs, and nuts. These foods are important sources of protein, calcium, iron, and zinc.

- This next level includes foods that come from plants—vegetables and fruits. Most people need to eat more of these foods for the vitamins, minerals, and fiber they supply.

- At the base of the pyramid are breads, cereals, rice, and pasta—all foods from grains. Most servings should come from these foods each day.

How Many Servings Do I Need?

The number of servings needed depends upon caloric need which is based on age, sex, size, and activity. Almost everyone needs at least the lowest number of servings in the ranges that are provided for each level. See Table 6-1 for sample diets at three calorie levels.

Table 6-1
Sample Diets for a Day at 3 Calorie Levels

	Women & some older adults	Children, teen girls, active women, most men	Teen boys & active men
Calorie level*	about 1600	about 2200	about 2800
Bread Group	6	9	11
Vegetable Group	3	4	5
Fruit Group	2	3	4
Milk Group	2–3	2–3	2–3
Meat Group (ounces)	5	6	7
Total Fat (grams)** (this amounts to 30% of calories)	53	73	93

* These are the calorie levels if you choose lowfat, lean foods from the 5 major food groups and use foods from the fats, oils, and sweets group sparingly.

** You can figure the number of grams of fat that provide 30% of calories in your daily diet as follows: multiply your daily calories by 0.30 (30 %) to get your calories from fat per day. For example **2200 calories x .30 = 660 calories from fat**; divide calories from fat per day by 9 (number of calories in a gram of fat) to get grams of fat per day. For example **660 calories from fat ÷ 9 = 73 grams of fat.** [1,2]

Source: U.S. Department of Agriculture/U.S. Department of Health and Human Services

What Is A Serving?

Many times, food is described by serving size, especially when counting the number of calories. The new food labeling has taken some of the guess work out of calorie counting, but what constitutes a serving is still a major question. Table 6-2 provides the answer.

Use the servings in Table 6-2 as a guide when selecting other foods not listed from the same food group. For mixed foods such as pizza or stew estimate the food group servings. For example, a generous serving of pizza would count in the bread group (crust), the milk group (the cheese), and the veg-

Table 6-2
What counts as a serving

Food Groups	
Bread, Cereal, Rice, and Pasta	6–11 Servings
1 slice of bread	
½ bun or bagel	
1 ounce of ready-to-eat cereal	
½ cup of cooked cereal, rice, pasta	
Vegetable	3–5 Servings
1 cup of raw leafy vegetables	
½ cup of other vegetables, cooked or chopped raw	
¾ cup of vegetable juice	
Fruit	2–4 Servings
1 medium apple, banana, orange, melon wedge	
½ cup of chopped, cooked or canned fruit	
¼ cup of dried fruit	
¾ cup of fruit juice	
Milk, Yogurt, Cheese	2–3 Servings
1 cup of milk (skim or low-fat)	
8 ounces low-fat yogurt	
1½ ounces of low-fat natural cheese	
2 ounces of low-fat processed cheese	
Meat, Poultry, Fish, Dry Beans, Eggs, and Nuts	2–3 Servings
2–3 ounces of cooked lean meat, poultry without skin, or fish	
½ cup of cooked dry beans	
1 egg or	
2 tablespoons of peanut butter counts as 1 ounce of lean meat (limit the use of egg yolks and organ meats since they are high in cholesterol).	

Source: *The Food Guide Pyramid.* U. S. Department of Agriculture. Home and Garden Bulletin #252.

etable group (the tomatoes, green peppers, etc.); a beef stew would count in the meat group and the vegetable group. Both have some fat as well.

MEALTIME STRATEGIES

Now that you have a basic understanding of the principles of a healthful diet, the question is how to put it all together when it comes to breakfast, lunch, and dinner. The following strategies are designed by the U.S. Department of Health and Human Services to improve your chances for a long and healthy life. By making the right food choices, the risk of developing cardiovascular disease and cancer may be reduced.

Breakfast
- *Strategy #1*—Choose fruit more often. Just a few great choices in the fruit family are cantaloupe, grapefruit, strawberries, oranges, bananas, pears, and apples.

- *Strategy #2*—Choose whole-grain cereals and products more often. Examples are whole wheat or bran breads, bagels, and cereal.

- *Strategy #3*—Try making pancakes and waffles with whole wheat flour instead of white flour and one whole egg and one egg white rather than two whole eggs. For a low-fat topping with fiber, try applesauce, apple butter and cinnamon, or fruit and low-fat plain yogurt.

- *Strategy #4*—Fruit juice and skim milk are familiar breakfast drinks. For an extra boost in the morning, why not try a fruit smoothie made from juice, fruit, and nonfat plain yogurt blended together. Other nonfat choices are seltzer water, coffee, and tea.

These low fat and low cholesterol breakfast choices provide good nutrition along with fiber, vitamins, and minerals. Some foods like sausage, bacon, butter, whole milk, and cream (including commercial nondairy creamer) should be chosen less often, because they are high in saturated fat and cholesterol.

Lunch
- *Strategy #1*—Try a fiber-rich bean, split pea, vegetable, or minestrone soup. Use commercially canned, frozen and cream soups less often—they can be high in sodium and fat. If you make your own soup, use broth or skim milk to keep the fat content low.

- *Strategy #2*—Try sandwiches made with water-packed tuna, sliced chicken, turkey, lean meat, or low-fat cheese, and use whole-grain bread or pita bread. To decrease fat, use reduced-calorie mayonnaise, just a SMALL AMOUNT of regular mayonnaise or mustard since it contains no fat.

- *Strategy #3*—Have a bean salad or mixed greens with plenty of vegetables. For fiber, include some vegetables like—carrots, broccoli, cauliflower, and kidney or garbanzo beans. For a low-fat dressing, try lemon juice or a reduced-calorie dressing. If you use regular dressing, use only a very small amount.

- *Strategy #4*—For dessert have fresh fruit, low-fat yogurt, or a frozen fruit bar.

- *Strategy #5*—Fruit juice and skim milk are good beverage choices. Club soda with a twist of lemon or lime, hot or iced tea with lemon, or coffee without cream are refreshing drinks.

Foods to eat less often include fried chicken, meat, or fish; processed luncheon meats; creamy salads; french fries and chips; rich or creamy desserts; high-fat baked goods; and high-fat cheeses such as swiss, cheddar, American, Brie.

Dinner
- *Strategy #1*—Eat a variety of vegetables. To increase variety, try some that might be new to you such as those from the cabbage family (broccoli, Brussels sprouts, cauliflower, and cabbage), dark-green leafy vegetables (spinach and kale), and yellow-orange vegetables (winter squash and sweet potatoes). For old favorites, like peas and green beans, skip the butter and sprinkle with lemon juice or herbs. Or how about a baked potato with the skin topped with low-fat yogurt and chives, tomato salsa, or a small amount of low-fat cheese?

- *Strategy #2*—Try whole wheat pasta and casseroles made with brown rice, bulgur, and other grains. If you are careful with preparation, these dishes can be excellent sources of fiber and low in fat. For example, when milk and eggs are ingredients in a recipe, try using one percent or skim milk, reduce the number of egg yolks and replace with egg whites. Here are some ideas for grain-based dishes:
  - whole-wheat spaghetti with fresh tomato sauce
  - whole wheat macaroni and chickpea stew in tomato sauce
  - tuna noodle casserole using water-packed tuna or rinsed, oil-packed tuna, skim milk, and fresh mushrooms or sliced water chestnuts
  - turkey, broccoli, and brown rice casserole using skim milk and egg whites
  - eggplant lasagna made with broiled eggplant and part-skim mozzarella or ricotta cheese
- *Strategy #3*—Substitute whole-grain breads and rolls for white bread
- *Strategy #4*—Choose main dishes that call for fish, chicken, turkey, or lean meat. Don't forget to remove the skin and visible fat from poultry and trim the fat from meat. Some good, low-fat choices are
  - red snapper stew
  - flounder or sole florentine (make the cream sauce with skim milk)
  - salmon loaf (use skim milk, rolled oats, and egg whites)
  - baked white fish with lemon and fennel
  - chicken cacciatore Italian-style (decrease the oil in the recipe)
  - chicken curry served over steamed wild rice (choose a recipe that requires little or no fat; "saute" the onions in chicken broth instead of butter)
  - light beef stroganoff with well-trimmed beef round steak and buttermilk served over noodles
  - oriental pork made with lean pork loin, green

peppers, and pineapple chunks served over rice

- *Strategy #5*—Choose desserts that give you fiber but little fat such as
  - baked apples or bananas sprinkled with cinnamon
  - fresh fruit cup
  - brown bread or rice pudding made with skim milk
  - oatmeal cookies (made with margarine or vegetable oil; add raisins)

Snacks

- *Strategy #1*—Try a raw vegetable platter made with a variety of vegetables. Include some good fiber choices such as carrots, snow peas, cauliflower, broccoli, and green beans.

- *Strategy #2*—Make sauces and dips with nonfat plain yogurt as the base.

- *Strategy #3*—Eat more fruit. Oranges, grapefruit, kiwi, apples, pears, bananas, strawberries, and cantaloupe are all good fiber sources. Make a big fruit salad and keep it on hand for snacks.

- *Strategy #4*—Plain, air-popped popcorn is a great low-fat snack with fiber. WATCH OUT! Some prepackaged microwave popcorn has fat added. Remember to go easy on the salt or use other seasonings.

- *Strategy #5*—Instead of chips try one of these low-fat alternatives that provide fiber—toasted shredded wheat squares sprinkled with a small amount of grated Parmesan cheese, whole-grain English muffins, or toasted plain corn tortillas.

- *Strategy #6*—When you are thirsty, try water, skim milk, juice, or club soda with a twist of lime or lemon.

Source: U.S. Department of Health and Human Services: National Cancer Institute and National Heart Lung and Blood Institute. *Eating for Life* (1988). NIH Publication No. 88-3000. Washington, DC: Superintendent of Documents U.S. Government Printing Office. U.S. Department of Agriculture & U.S. Department of Health and Human Services (1990). *Dietary Guidelines for Americans* (3rd ed.). Home and Garden Bulletin No. 232.

THE "NEW FOOD LABEL"

Shopping for food can be an awesome task if you are attempting to break down all purchases into their appropriate food groups, especially processed foods. Grocery shopping need not be such a burden. As of May 1994, food manufacturers have begun labeling their products in compliance with the 1990 Nutrition Labeling and Education Act. The food label helps consumers choose a healthier diet and offers an incentive to food companies to improve the nutritional quality of their products. See Figure 6-2.

Nutrition Facts

Serving Size 1 cup (228g)
Servings Per Container 2

Amount Per Serving

Calories 260 Calories from Fat 120

	% Daily Values*
Total Fat 13g	20%
Saturated Fat 5g	25%
Cholesterol 30 mg	10%
Sodium 660 mg	28%
Total Carbohydrate 31g	10%
Dietary Fiber 0g	0%
Sugars 5g	
Protein 5g	

Vitamin A 4%	•	Vitamin C 2%
Calcium 15%	•	Iron 4%

*Percent Daily Values are based on a 2,000 calorie diet. Your daily values may be higher or lower depending on your calorie needs:

		Calories	2,000	2,500
Total Fat	Less than		65g	80g
Sat Fat	Less than		20g	25g
Cholesterol	Less than		300mg	300mg
Sodium	Less than		2,400mg	2,400mg
Total Carbohydrates			300g	375g
Dietary Fiber			25g	30g

Calories per gram:
Fat 9 • Carbohydrate 4 • Protein 4

Source: FDA Medical Bulletin May 94. Volume 24 Number 1.
Department of Health and Human Service. Rockville, Maryland

Figure 6-2
The "New Food Label"

Fresh Foods

Even fresh foods are not a problem. Nutrition information for the 20 most commonly eaten raw fruits and vegetables and 20 most commonly eaten types of fresh seafood is now available to consumers in grocery stores in the appropriate departments. This information may be found on posters, shelf labels, or in brochures. In addition, nutrition information appears on over 90% of processed packaged foods.

Exempt Foods

Foods that are exempt from this labeling process are plain coffee and tea; some spices, flavorings, and foods containing no significant amounts of nutrients; ready-to-eat deli and bakery items prepared on site; restaurant food; bulk food that is not resold; and food produced by small businesses. Also food that is in small packages (breath mints, meat or poultry products less than half an ounce) is not required to carry the new label.

Serving Size Information

The information on the food label is usually expressed by individual serving size. The serving size is realistic and consistent across product lines to make comparisons easier.

Nutritional Claims

Marketing strategies have always tried to make us believe one product was better than another. When it comes to nutrition, what companies are able to say is highly controlled. Nutrition claims such as "free," "low," "light," "reduced," "less," or "high" have to meet FDA definitions. Each definition now means the same thing from one product to another. See Table 6-3.

What Some Claims Mean   If labels make certain health claims, they must be based on scientific fact. The FDA has approved claims on labels that certain nutrients may act to prevent particular diseases. These claims connect the following nutrients to their related diseases

- calcium to osteoporosis
- fiber-containing grain products, fruits, and vegetables to cancer
- fruits, vegetables, and grain products that contain fiber to coronary heart disease
- fat to cancer
- saturated fat and cholesterol to coronary heart disease
- sodium to hypertension

Source: Department of Health and Human Services. Public Health Service. Food and Drug Administration. *FDA Medical Bulletin*, May'94, Volume 24, Number 1.

Table 6-3
New Food Label: What Some Claims Mean

High Protein	At least 10 grams (g) high-quality protein per serving
Good Source of Calcium	At least 100 milligrams (mg) calcium per serving
More Iron	At least 1.8 mg more iron per serving than reference food.* (Label will say 10 percent more of the Daily Value for iron.)
Fat-Free	Less than 0.5 g fat per serving
Low-Fat	3 g or less fat per serving.
Reduced Calories	At least 25 percent fewer calories per serving than the reference food*
Sugar-Free	Less than 0.5 g sugar per serving
Light (two meanings)	One-third fewer calories or half the fat of the reference food.* (If 50 percent or more of the food's calories are from fat, the fat must be reduced by 50 percent)
	A "low-calorie, "low-fat" food whose calorie/fat content has been reduced by 50 percent of the reference food*

*Reference food is food that the "claim" product is compared to, e.g., lite fruit cocktail to fruit cocktail in heavy syrup.
Source: Food Label Makes Good Eating Easier by P. Kurtzweil, 1995, *FDA Consumer.* The Magazine of the U.S. Food and Drug Administration, 29 (7) p. 19. DHHS Publication No. (FDA) 95-1001. Superintendent of Documents: Pittsburgh, PA.

MAINTAIN HEALTHY WEIGHT

Being overweight is a common condition in the United States. Overweight and obese conditions are associated with high blood pressure, heart disease, stroke, the most common type of diabetes, certain cancers, and other types of illness.

Whether your weight is "healthy" depends on how much of your weight is fat, where in your body the fat is located, and whether there are weight-related medical problems.

What Is A Healthy Weight?
What is a healthy weight for you? Right now there is no exact answer to an individual's healthy weight, but scientists are actively working to develop more precise measurement methods. Figure 6-3 will help you determine whether your weight is "healthy."

Weight Range
Weights above the healthy weight range are generally believed to be unhealthy for most people. The further you are above the healthy weight range for your height, the higher your risk. Weights slightly below the range may be healthy for some people but are sometimes the result of health problems, especially when weight loss is not intentional.

Body Shape And Weight
In addition to weight, another factor which affects health is body shape. Excess fat located in the abdominal area (apple-shape) as opposed to the hips and thighs (pear-shape) poses a greater health risk. To check your body shape:

- measure around your waist near your navel while you stand relaxed, not pulling in your abdomen
- measure around your hips, over the buttocks, where they are largest
- divide the waist measurement by the hip measurement to calculate your waist-to-hip ratio. Ratios close to or above ONE are linked with greater risk. For example a person with a 30 inch waist and 42 inch hips (30 ÷ 42 = 0.7) has more of a pear-shaped body than someone with a 40 inch waist and 36 inch hips (40 ÷ 36 = 1) who has an apple-shaped body.

If weight and the waist-to-hip ratio are acceptable and no medical problems exist, then no weight change is needed. If

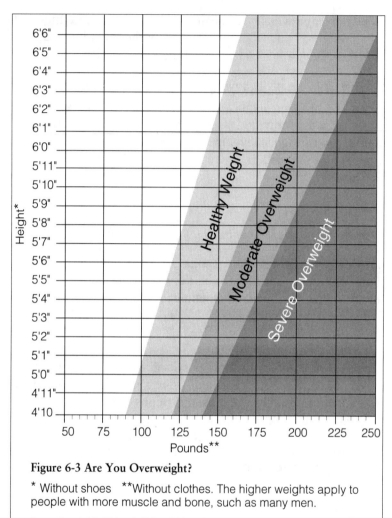

Figure 6-3 Are You Overweight?

* Without shoes   **Without clothes. The higher weights apply to people with more muscle and bone, such as many men.

Source: Report of the Dietary Guidelines Advisory Committee on the Dietary Guidelines for Americans. 1995. pages 23–24. Fourth edition, 1995. U.S. Department of Agriculture. U.S. Department of Health and Human Services.

you have any questions, or the ranges for waist-to-hip ratio and/or weight cause you to be concerned, seek the attention of your health care provider.[1,2]

What If I Want to Lose Weight?

The Facts About Weight Loss
- Any claims that you can lose weight effortlessly are false. The weight-loss business is a booming industry. Americans spend an estimated $30 billion a year on all types of diet programs and products including diet foods and drinks. Trying to sort out all of the competing claims—often misleading, unproven, or just plain false—can be confusing and costly.

  Weight loss is a simple formula—the body must use more calories than it consumes. When diet specialists talk about the body using calories, they may also say "burn" or "metabolize" calories. The question becomes "What is the best way to accomplish this?" Rather than severely restricting caloric intake and depressing the body's ability to use calories, weight-loss specialists now advise moderate exercise as a means of achieving weight control. "A person not only burns calories while exercising, but if he or she is eating an adequate amount of food, calories will continue to be burned at a higher rate for up to several hours afterward.[2] For most people, cutting fat intake and adding moderate exercise can work as well as a commercial weight control program.

  Exercisers are also more likely than sedentary people to keep weight off, whether they use a "do-it-yourself" diet or attend a program. The only proven way to lose weight is either to reduce the number of calories you eat or to increase the number of calories you burn off through exercise. Most experts recommend a combination of both. As a matter of fact, when diet alone is used in a weight reduction program, weight is usually regained, whereas diet combined with exercise leads to better maintenance. Several studies have shown that regular exercise is a central component in losing weight and is the single best predictor of long-term weight maintenance.[3]

- Fad diets rarely have any permanent effect. Sudden and radical changes in your eating patterns are difficult to sustain over time. In addition, so-called "crash" diets often send dieters into a cycle of quick weight loss, followed by a "rebound" weight gain once normal eating resumes. The weight will be even more difficult to lose the next time a diet is attempted.

- Very low-calorie diets, usually less than 1000 calories, are not without risk and should be pursued only under medical supervision. Unsupervised very low-calorie diets can deprive you of important nutrients and are potentially dangerous. Furthermore, these very restricted calorie diets tell your body that, essentially, it is starving. Your body adjusts by lowering its metabolism and holding onto the body fat you had hoped to lose.

  Many times there will be initial quick weight loss, which is mostly fluid with little actual weight loss.

- To lose weight safely and keep it off requires long-term changes in daily eating and exercise habits. Many experts recommend a goal of losing about a pound a week. A modest reduction of 500 calories per day will allow you to achieve this goal, since a total reduction of 3,500 calories is required to lose one pound of fat.

  Reducing your caloric consumption by 500 calories a day is not needed if exercise is added to the weight reduction program. Table 6-4 shows ways to increase your calorie expenditure.[4,5]

Calories In spite of all the hundreds of reducing diets that have been around for years and seem to appear regularly, the best and simplest way to lose weight is to increase physical activity and reduce the fat and sugars in the diet. Since fat is a high calorie item, reducing fat in the diet automatically cuts down on the number of calories consumed. Fat has more than twice the calories as the same amount of protein or carbohydrate. Protein and carbohydrate both have about four calories in each gram, but all fat—saturated, polyunsaturated, or monounsaturated—has nine calories in each gram. Thus, foods that are high in fat are high in calories. And all calories count, so to maintain a desirable weight, it is important to eat no more calories than your body needs.

Burning Calories Calories are only half the equation of weight control. Physical activity burns calories, increases the proportion of lean to fat body mass, and raises your metabolism. Thus, a combination of both is important for success.

Table 6-4
Calorie Values for 10 Minutes of Activity

Activity	Body Weight		
	125 Pounds	175 Pounds	250 Pounds
Personal Necessities			
Sleeping	10	14	20
Sitting (Watching TV)	10	14	18
Sitting (Talking)	15	21	30
Dressing or Washing	26	37	53
Standing	12	16	24
Locomotion			
Walking Downstairs	56	78	111
Walking Upstairs	146	202	288
Walking at 2 mph	29	40	58
Walking at 4 mph	52	72	102
Running at 5.5 mph	90	125	178
Running at 7 mph	118	164	232
Running at 12 mph	164	228	326
Cycling at 5.5 mph	42	58	83
Cycling at 13 mph	89	124	178
Housework			
Making Beds	32	46	65
Washing Floors	38	53	75
Washing Windows	35	48	69
Dusting	22	31	44
Preparing a Meal	32	46	65
Shoveling Snow	65	89	130
Light Gardening	30	42	59
Weeding Garden	49	68	98
Mowing Grass (manual)	38	52	74
Mowing Grass (power)	34	47	67
Sedentary Occupation			
Sitting Writing	15	21	30
Light Office Work	25	34	50
Standing, Light Activity	20	28	40
Typing (Electric)	19	27	39
Light Work			
Assembly Line	20	28	40
Auto Repair	35	48	69
Carpentry	32	44	64
Bricklaying	28	40	57
Farming Chores	32	44	64
House Painting	29	40	58

(continued)

Table 6-4
Calorie Values for 10 Minutes of Activity *(continued)*

Activity	Body Weight		
	125 Pounds	175 Pounds	250 Pounds
Heavy Work			
Pick & Shovel Work	56	78	110
Chopping Wood	60	84	121
Dragging Logs	158	220	315
Drilling Coal	79	111	159
Recreation			
Badminton	43	65	94
Baseball	39	54	78
Basketball	58	82	117
Bowling (nonstop)	56	78	111
Canoeing (4 mph)	90	128	182
Dancing (moderate)	35	48	69
Dancing (vigorous)	48	66	94
Football	69	96	137
Golfing	33	48	68
Horseback Riding	56	78	112
Ping-Pong	32	45	64
Racquetball	75	104	144
Skiing (Alpine)	80	112	160
Skiing (Cross Country)	98	138	194
Skiing (Water)	60	88	130
Squash	75	104	144
Swimming (backstroke)	32	45	64
Swimming (crawl)	40	56	80
Tennis	56	80	115
Volleyball	43	65	94

The best way to determine whether all of this is working is to "keep stepping on the scale."

Decreasing Calories   To decrease calorie intake, eat a variety of foods low in calories and high in nutrients. It is important to

• eat less fat and fatty foods

- eat more fruits, vegetables; breads and cereals—without fats and sugars added in preparation or at the table
- eat less sugars and sweets
- drink little or no alcoholic beverages
- eat smaller portions and limit second helpings
- avoid diets of less than 1200 calories because they lack the daily requirements for a healthy diet; and
- develop new exercise and eating habits to promote interest and achieve success

CHOOSE A DIET LOW IN FAT, SATURATED FAT, AND CHOLESTEROL

Most health authorities recommend an American diet with less fat, saturated fat, and cholesterol. A diet low in fat makes it easier to include the variety of food you need for nutrients without exceeding your calorie needs, because fat contains over twice the calories of an equal amount of carbohydrates or protein.

The way diet affects cholesterol varies among individuals. However, blood cholesterol does increase in most people when they eat a diet high in saturated fat, cholesterol, and excessive calories. For a diet low in fat, saturated fat, and cholesterol see Chapter 5.

CHOOSE A DIET WITH PLENTY OF VEGETABLES, FRUITS, AND GRAIN PRODUCTS

Vegetables, fruits, and grain products are important parts of a varied diet and are emphasized here, especially for their complex carbohydrates, dietary fiber, and other food components linked to good health. These foods are generally low in fats. By choosing the recommended servings in the "Food Guide Pyramid," carbohydrates will most likely increase and fat intake will decrease. Intake of dietary fiber will also increase.

Populations such as ours with diets low in dietary fiber and complex carbohydrates and high in fat, especially saturated fat, tend to have more heart disease, obesity, and some cancer. Complex carbohydrates, such as starches, are found in breads, cereals, pasta, rice, dry beans and peas, and other vegetables such as potatoes and corn. Just how dietary fiber is involved in the healthy diet is not yet clear. Some of the benefit may come from the food that provides the fiber, not from fiber alone. For this reason, it is best to get fiber from foods rather than from supplements. Furthermore, excessive use of fiber supplements is associated with greater risk for intestinal problems and lower absorption of some minerals. Dietary fiber—a part of plant foods—is in whole-grain breads and cereals, dry beans and peas, vegetables, and fruits. It is best to eat a variety of these fiber-rich foods, because they differ in the kinds of fiber they contain.

USE SUGARS ONLY IN MODERATION

What are "sugars"? Common sugars are listed below.

- Table sugar (sucrose)
- Brown sugar
- Raw sugar
- Glucose (dextrose)
- Maltose
- Molasses
- Fruit juice concentrate
- Honey
- Syrup
- Corn sweetener
- Fructose

- Corn syrup
- Lactose

Read food labels, since a food is likely to be high in sugar if its ingredient list shows one of the sugars first or second, or if it shows several of them. Americans eat sugar in many forms.

Sugar provides calories and most people like its taste. The problem with many foods is that they contain large amounts of sugar and lots of calories which can increase weight, and unfortunately these calories are often limited in nutrients. Calories which supply no benefit to the body are called "empty calories." Thus, they should be used in moderation by most healthy people. Sugars and starches, which breakdown into sugar, are found in many foods which also supply nutrients—milk, fruit, some vegetables, breads, cereals, and other foods. Because of the high sugar content, the more often these foods—even small amounts—are eaten, and the longer they are in the mouth before teeth are brushed, the greater the risk for tooth decay.

Diabetes is a disorder which causes sugar to build up in the blood. Diets high in sugar have not been shown to cause diabetes. The most common type of diabetes occurs in overweight adults, and simply avoiding sugar will not correct overweight problems.

USE SALT AND SODIUM ONLY IN MODERATION

Table salt contains sodium and chloride—both of which are essential in the diet. However, most Americans eat more salt and sodium than they need. Food and beverages containing salt provide most of the sodium in our diets, much of it added during processing and manufacturing.

In populations with diets low in salt, high blood pressure is less common than in populations with diets high in salt. Other factors that affect blood pressure are heredity, obesity, and excessive drinking of alcoholic beverages.

Some people who do not have high blood pressure may reduce their risk of getting it by eating a diet with less salt and other sources of sodium. At present, there is no way to predict who might develop high blood pressure and who will benefit from reducing dietary salt and sodium. However, it is wise for most people to eat less salt and sodium, because for the most part they need much less than they eat and a reduction in salt will benefit those people whose blood pressure rises with salt intake. Since more than half of all women over the age of 55 have high blood pressure, a decreased salt intake makes a great deal of sense!

Salt and sodium intake includes the salt or sodium already contained in the food plus whatever is added during cooking and at the table. Total sodium intake should not exceed 2400 milligrams daily. To moderate the use of salt and sodium, follow the advice below.

- use salt sparingly, if at all, in cooking and at the table
- when planning meals, consider that
  - fresh and plain frozen vegetables prepared without salt are lower in sodium than canned ones
  - cereals, pasta, and rice cooked without salt are lower in sodium than ready-to-eat cereals;
  - milk and yogurt are lower in sodium than most cheeses
  - fresh meat, poultry, and fish are lower in sodium than most canned and processed ones
  - most frozen dinners and combination dishes, packaged mixes, canned soups, and salad dressings contain a considerable amount of sodium as do condiments, such as soy and other sauces, pickles, olives, catsup, and mustard
- use salted snacks, such as chips, crackers, pretzels, and nuts, sparingly
- check labels for the amount of sodium in foods and choose those lower in sodium most of the time.

Source: U.S. Department of Health and Human Services: National Cancer Institute and National Heart Lung and Blood Institute. *Eating for Life* (1988). NIH Publication No. 88-3000. Washington, DC: Superintendent of Documents U.S. Government Printing Office.

IF YOU DRINK ALCOHOLIC BEVERAGES, DO SO IN MODERATION

Alcoholic beverages supply calories, but little or no nutrients. Most drinks contain 100-200 calories each. Drinking alcohol is linked with many health problems, is the cause of many accidents, and can lead to addiction.

Women who are trying to control their weight may want to cut down on alcohol and substitute calorie-free iced tea, mineral water, or seltzer with a squeeze of lemon or lime.

Over the last several years, a number of studies have reported that moderate drinkers—those who have one or two drinks per day—are less likely to develop heart disease than people who don't drink any alcohol. If you are a nondrinker, this is not a recommendation to start using alcohol since drinking alcoholic beverages may raise blood pressure which could lead to stroke. In the face of such conflicting information, it is well-known that people who drink heavily on a regular basis have higher rates of heart disease than either moderate drinkers or nondrinkers.

For those of you who do enjoy alcoholic beverages, moderation is the key. Heavy drinking can definitely cause heart-related problems. More than two drinks per day can raise blood pressure, and recent research shows that binge drinking can lead to stroke.

What Is Moderate Drinking? For women, "moderate drinking" is no more than one drink per day, according to the U.S. Dietary Guidelines for Americans. Count as one drink

- 12 ounces of beer

- 5 ounces of wine

- 1½ ounces of hard liquor (80 proof)

Source: *Dietary Guidelines for Americans*, U.S. Department of Agriculture/U.S. Department of Health and Human Services, 1990.

ANTIOXIDANTS

The possibility of a relationship between diet and disease has been a major preoccupation of scientists throughout history. Increasing evidence that antioxidant vitamins protect against a number of diseases, including heart disease, cataracts and serious age-related eye disease which can lead to blindness, and certain types of cancer, has prompted an interest in the action of antioxidants.

How Do They Work?

How do antioxidants work? Oxidation is the combination of a substance with oxygen which causes a breakdown or change in the substance. Antioxidants are defense systems that provide protection against oxidative damage to tissue. For example, the oxidation of LDL can affect factors which may lead to heart disease. If antioxidants inhibit the oxidation of LDL, then atherosclerosis (a common form of arteriosclerosis in which deposits of yellowish plaque containing cholesterol and other fatty deposits adhere to the blood vessel walls), can be prevented or slowed.

Vitamins And Carotenoids

The main antioxidant vitamins are vitamin C, E, and beta carotene (pro-vitamin A). Beta carotene is not actually a vitamin, but is commonly included in the "antioxidant vitamin group." Beta carotene is but one of a large group of carotenoids with antioxidant activity. Carotenoids are simply a group of pigments, yellow to deep red in color, consisting of certain hydrogen and carbon substances which concentrate in animal fat when eaten. Carotenoids play an important role in nature by protecting cells and organisms and are found predominantly in fruits and vegetables. Carrots are a primary source of beta carotene. Other carotenoids with antioxidant activity include lycopene, lutein, and zeaxanthin in tomatoes, spinach, and collard greens.

Skepticism

Early interest was generated in carotenoids when it was found that consumers of fruits and vegetables, especially green and yellow leafy vegetables, had a reduced risk of cancer. Beta carotene was the primary focus, because it was the best known and because it also has potential vitamin A activity.

Research

After a long history of optimistic reports about these dietary antioxidants, some recent reports have caused skepticism. The controversy actually has merit since it has pointed out that not all antioxidants are the same, and antioxidants differ in their ability to prevent certain diseases. In other words, if one antioxidant is not effective, it does not mean they are all ineffective.

Women's Health Study

Much of this research is relatively new. It appears antioxidants have a role to play and until more conclusive data is available the most prudent recommendation is that we do those things that we know will reduce our risk of heart disease, cancer, and eye disorders which includes eating a well-balanced diet high in fruits and vegetables.[6,7,8,9,10]

Of particular interest to women will be the "Women's Health Study," a five-year study of 40,000 postmenopausal women which began in 1992. It is the first clinical trial conducted on women using beta carotene and vitamin E. Benefits and risks of taking beta carotene, low doses of aspirin, and vitamin E to prevent cancer and cardiovascular disease will be evaluated. Although the focus is on heart disease and cancer risk factors, other questions about breast implants, tissue disorders, breast cancer, and the relationship of aspirin to migraine prevention will also be examined.[11,12]

EXERCISE

Most Americans get little vigorous exercise at work or during leisure hours. People usually ride in cars or buses and watch

TV during their free time rather than being physically active. Activities like bowling provide some benefit, but they do not provide the same benefits as regular, more vigorous exercise. Evidence suggests that even low- to moderate-intensity activities can have both short- and long-term benefits.[13]

Benefits

Many people who exercise find that they wake up more rested and look forward to the day ahead. Besides the physical benefits of exercise, the psychological benefits are recognizable. A person who looks good, and appears mentally alert will appear to be in command of their life. A sense of well-being and self pride in a goal achieved emanates from a healthy individual. Exercising regularly is not always easy, but the rewards are great![14]

The value of exercise in the prevention of osteoporosis, cardiovascular disease, and other problems encountered during the menopause transition was discussed earlier. Remember, regular physical activity lowers the risk of high blood pressure, diabetes, and breast and colon cancer. It makes you

Feel Better
- gives you more energy
- helps you cope with stress
- improves your self-image
- increases resistance to fatigue
- helps counter anxiety and depression
- helps you to relax and feel less tense
- improves the ability to fall asleep quickly and sleep well
- provides an easy way to share an activity with friends or family and an opportunity to meet new friends

Look Better
- tones your muscles

- has a beneficial effect on flexibility and coordination
- burns off calories to help lose extra pounds or help you stay at your desirable weight
- helps control your appetite

Work Better
- helps you to be more productive at work
- increases your capacity for physical work
- builds stamina for other physical activities
- increases muscle strength
- helps your heart and lungs work more efficiently

Source: *Exercise and Your Heart: A Guide to Physical Activity.* (1993). (Rev. ed). National Institutes of Health. National Heart, Lung and Blood Institute. American Heart Association. (NIH Publication No. 93-1677). Washington, D.C.: U.S. Government Printing Office.

Circulation

When estrogen levels decrease there seems to be a reduction in blood flow to every part of the body. Regular exercise will increase the strength and function of the whole body as well as increase the general circulation of blood throughout the body.

Never Too Young Nor Too Old For Exercise

Exercise can play an important role in ensuring an appropriate quality of life in middle age and later, but to be most effective, it needs to start at an earlier age, preferably during the premenopausal period of a woman's life. Consider it safe to say for the purposes of this discussion, the premenopausal period starts during childhood! It is never too early to start some kind of an exercise program especially when it is reported that children and adolescents are watching too much television and exercising less. Today one in five teens is overweight, which is no doubt partly responsible for the startlingly high numbers of overweight individuals in the United States.

However, it is never too late to start some kind of an exercise program, for a "lack of activity does more harm than good, both physically and mentally."

Five Common Myths About Exercise

Myth 1. Exercising makes you tired. As people become more physically fit, most feel that physical activity gives them even more energy than before. Regular, moderate-to-brisk exercise can also help to reduce fatigue and manage stress.

Myth 2. Exercising takes too much time. Regular exercise for 30 to 60 minutes three or four times a week is all that is needed to CONDITION your heart and lungs. If you have difficulty finding 30 minutes in your schedule for an exercise break, try to find two 15-minutes periods or even three 10-minute periods.

Myth 3. All exercises give you the same benefits. All physical activities can give enjoyment plus many other benefits which have already been described, but only regular, brisk, and sustained exercises such as brisk walking, jogging, or swimming improve the efficiency of your heart and lungs and burn off substantial extra calories.

Myth 4. The older you are the less exercise you need. As individuals age, they become less active. In general middle-aged and older people benefit from regular physical activity just as young people do. Age should not be a limitation. Actually, regular physical activity in older persons increases their capacity to perform activities of daily living. What is most important is tailoring the activity program to a personal fitness level. Even individuals with arthritis and other conditions which interfere with movement can benefit from exercise. Usually the pain of these ailments prevents any type of exercise. Inactivity often compounds the problem; "If you don't use it, you lose it." If you are affected by any of these diseases which restrict your movements, check first with your health care provider before embarking on any kind of an exercise program.

Myth 5. You have to be athletic to exercise. Special athletic skills are not required for most physical activities. Many of these activities are easy to do and require no special talent or athletic ability. Walking is a perfect example.

Source: *Exercise and Your Heart: A Guide to Physical Activity.* (1993). (Rev. ed.). National Institutes of Health. National Heart, Lung and Blood Institute. American Heart Association. (NIH Publication No. 93-1677). Washington, D.C.: U.S. Government Printing Office.

What Kind Of Exercise Program Is Best?

Admittedly, the management of a career, an exercise program, and maybe even a family seems like a difficult task. The key to success is choosing an activity (or activities) that you enjoy. A well-rounded program combines aerobic exercise for cardiovascular conditioning with exercises for flexibility, muscle strengthening, bone density, and relaxation. Likewise, any program undertaken should be one that is satisfying and fulfilling, not painful or boring.

Exercise Outdoors Or In Your Home?

Don't think you need fancy equipment or a health club or class to exercise. The home environment can supply plenty of exercise opportunity. Videos and television exercise programs combined with space-saving devices and other activities can make for a varied, successful, healthy workout which will benefit your muscles, bones, and heart.

Enthusiasts who like outdoor activities such as biking, tennis, walking, or jogging need rainy- or snow-day back-up plans to stay on a regular schedule. For these days, stationary cycling, bench stepping, running in place, or jumping rope can be good alternatives in addition to using some of the equipment that is readily available at almost any price and for almost any type of space. Make certain that routines vary to prevent boredom and to work different body parts.

Do You Like To Exercise Alone Or With Other People?

Exercise activities can be performed alone, with a partner, or in a group. All three can be inviting and helpful. Some people prefer companionship to get started and to keep going.

Others enjoy the peace and quiet of a private workout. For those who have difficulty staying with a program at home, many community and health clubs offer inexpensive, professional aerobics. Whatever works best for you is most important. Choose an activity that is enjoyable and one that will fit most easily into your schedule AND STAY WITH IT!

What Is The Best Fit Between Activity And Schedule?

An exercise routine should most definitely be a scheduled activity. The act of creating a schedule affirms your commitment. Whether the activity occurs in the morning, afternoon, or evening makes little difference as long as it is accomplished. A realistic schedule coupled with activities that are enjoyed ensures their ongoing place in your day.

Exercise is for everyone and you do not have to train like a marathon runner to become more physically fit! Age doesn't matter. The difference exercise can make is easy to see.

Do I Need A Complete Physical Examination Before I Start?

Most people do not need to see a doctor or other health professionals before they start a gradual, sensible exercise program. Some people, however, should get medical advice. An examination is warranted if current health problems exist (especially heart trouble), if one is over 50 years old and is not used to energetic activity, or if a family history of heart disease developing at a young age exists. Joint, back, or muscle problems; illness; or disabilities call for a discussion with a health professional.

Where Do I Begin?

Build up slowly. If you have been inactive for a long while, time will be needed to get into shape. Start with low- to moderate-level activities for at least several minutes each day.

For those who want to start an activity program and do not know how or where to begin, two examples can be found in Appendix A, walking and jogging programs. Walking and jogging programs are easy ways for most people to get regular exercise, because they don't require special facilities or equipment other than good, comfortable shoes and proper dress for the weather.

Effective Ways To Avoid Problems

- Try not to set your goals too high once you start an exercise program or you may push yourself too far too quickly.

- Before each exercise session, allow a 5-minute period of stretching and slow exercise to give your body a chance to "warm up." At the end of your workout, take another 5 minutes to "cool down" with a slower, less energetic exercise pace.

- Listen to your body. A certain amount of stiffness is normal at first, but if you hurt a joint or muscle, stop exercising for several days to avoid more serious injury. There is no truth to the old saying "no pain, no gain"! Start slowly and build up. Do a little less than you think you can at first. Later, when you know your limits, do more.

- Be aware of possible signs of heart problems such as

  - pain or pressure in the chest area, left neck, shoulder, or arm during or just after exercising or

  - sudden lightheadedness, cold sweat, pallor, or fainting.

- Should any of these signals occur, stop exercising and seek medical attention immediately.

- Take appropriate precautions during special weather conditions.

  - On hot, humid days

    - exercise during the cooler and/or less humid parts of the day such as early morning or early evening

    - exercise less than normal for a week until you become accustomed to the heat

    - drink lots of fluids, especially water before,

during, and after exercising (extra salt is not usually needed because enough salt is in the diet)

- watch out for signs of heat stroke—feeling dizzy, weak, light-headed, and/or excessively tired; sweating stops; or body temperature becomes dangerously high

- wear a minimum of loose-fitting clothing

- avoid rubberized or plastic suits and sweat pants which can cause dangerously high temperatures, possibly resulting in heat stroke

- On cold days

  - wear one layer less than if you were not exercising or wear several layers rather than one heavy layer, so you can remove one if you get too warm

  - wear mittens, gloves, or old socks; and

  - wear a hat, since up to 40 percent of your body's heat is lost through your neck and head.[13]

WALKING

Walking is often dismissed as being "too easy," but studies show that, when done briskly on a regular schedule, it can improve the body's ability to consume oxygen during exertion, lower the resting heart rate, reduce blood pressure, and increase the efficiency of the heart and lungs. Walking also helps burn excess calories, and has some unique advantages.

- Almost everyone can do it. You don't have to take lessons. All you need to become a serious walker is to increase your pace and distance and walk more often. When you're walking for exercise, you don't saunter, stroll, or shuffle. You move out at a steady clip that is brisk enough to make your heart beat faster and cause you to breathe more deeply

- You can walk almost anywhere. Almost any SAFE sidewalk, street, road, trail, park, field, or shopping mall will do.

- You can walk almost anytime. You can set your own schedule since you do not really need a partner or a team. For the most part, weather is not as much of a problem as it is with other kinds of activities as long as you are dressed appropriately.

Warm-up And Conditioning Exercises

Although walking is good exercise for the legs, heart, lungs and backbone, it does not improve upper body tone or strength. Therefore some "WARM-UP exercises" follow which will increase your flexibility and strength and should always be done before walking. Upper body exercises in Figure 3-9 can also be used as part of a "Warm Up" program.

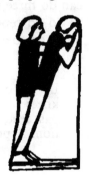

Stretcher   Stand facing a wall, an arms' length away. Lean forward and place palms of hands flat against wall, slightly below shoulder height. Keep back straight, heels firmly on floor, and slowly bend elbows until forehead touches wall. Tuck hips toward wall and hold position for 20 seconds. **Repeat exercise with knees slightly flexed.**

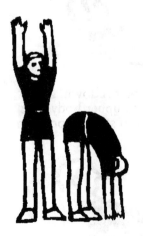

Reach And Bend   Stand erect with feet shoulder-width apart and arms extended over the head. Reach as high as possible while keeping heels on floor and hold for 10 counts. Flex knees slightly and bend slowly at waist, touching floor between feet with fingers. Hold for 10 counts (if you cannot touch the floor, try to touch the tops of your shoes.) **Repeat entire sequence 2 to 5 times.**

Knee Pull
Lie flat on back with legs extended
and arms at sides. Lock arms
around legs just below knees and
pull knees to chest, raising buttocks slightly off floor. Hold for 10
to 15 counts. (If you have knee
problems, you may find it easier to
lock arms behind knees.) **Repeat
exercise 3 to 5 times.**

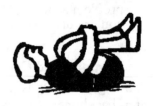

Situp Several versions of the situp are listed (easiest one listed first, most difficult one last). Start with the situp that you
can do three times without undue strain. When you are able
to do 10 repetitions of the exercise without great difficulty,
move on to a more difficult version.

- Lie flat on back with arms at sides, palms down, and
  knees slightly bent. Curl head forward until you can see
  past feet, hold for three counts, then lower to start position. **Repeat exercise 3 to 10 times.**

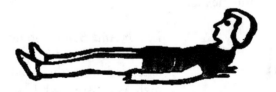

- Lie flat on back with arms at sides, palms down, and
  knees slightly bent. Roll forward until upper body is at
  45-degree angle to floor, then return to starting position.
  Repeat exercise 3 to 10 times.

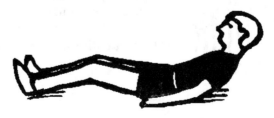

- Lie flat on back with arms at sides, palms down, and knees slightly bent. Roll forward to sitting position, then return to starting position. **Repeat exercise 3 to 10 times.**

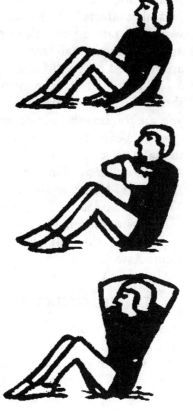

- Lie flat on back with arms crossed on chest and knees slightly bent. Roll forward to sitting position. Then return to starting position. **Repeat exercise 3 to 10 times.**

- Lie flat on back with hands laced in back of head and knees slightly bent. Roll forward to sitting position, then return to starting position. **Repeat exercise 3 to 15 times.**

Source: *Walking for Exercise and Pleasure*. (1992). The President's Council on Physical Fitness and Sports GPO: 1992 0-326-101. Washington, DC: Superintendent of Documents, U.S. Government.

How Far? How Fast? How Soon? If you have been living a fairly sedentary life for a number of years, you may be shocked at how poor your condition is. You can systematically build up your stamina and strength with time. No one knows exactly how far or how fast you should walk when beginning a walking program. It is best to begin walking 20 minutes at least four or five times a week at a pace that feels comfortable. If too tiring, then reduce the pace or length of time. As your condition improves, you should gradually increase your time and pace. Eventually, the goal should be to get to the place where you can comfortably walk three miles in 45 minutes, but there is no need to rush to get there.

It takes about 20 minutes for your body to begin realizing the "training effects" of sustained exercise. The more often you walk, the faster you will improve. Three workouts a week are considered "maintenance level," more frequent workouts are required for swift improvement.

The "talk test" can help you find the right pace. You should be able to carry on a conversation while walking. If you are too breathless, you are going too fast.

Some experts say that it takes a month of reconditioning to make up for each year of physical inactivity. See Appendix A for a sample walking program and jogging program.[15] The American Heart Association has a brochure entitled "Walking...Natural Fun, Natural Fitness" with a walking readiness questionnaire and a one-mile fitness test. You can request this through your local chapter of the American Heart Association.

AEROBIC EXERCISE

Only regular, sustained, brisk exercise will improve heart and lung health. This is called "aerobic" exercise and some of the more vigorous exercises include jogging, swimming, jumping rope, cross-country skiing, stair climbing, walking briskly, and bicycling. Aerobic exercises should be performed for at least 30 minutes, three or four times a week, at more than 50% of your exercise capacity. See Table 6-5. Walking moderately, tennis (singles), volleyball, downhill skiing, and dancing can also strengthen your heart, if you do them fast enough and for 30 minutes or longer, three to four times a week.

Target Heart Rate Zone

Keeping track of your heart rate during exercise is important. Your heart should beat faster when exercising. How fast it should beat depends on age. Each person has a heart rate target zone. The number of heartbeats per minute should fall within the target zone to make exercise worthwhile. It is important to reach and maintain the target zone to condition the heart. Working out above the target zone is too hard on the heart. Exercise below 50% gives the heart and lungs little conditioning. Therefore, the best activity level is 50 to 75% of this maximum rate. The 50-75% range is called the TARGET HEART RATE ZONE. The maximum heart rate is approximately 220 minus your age. Find your target zone in Table 6-5.

Table 6–5
Target Heart Rate
(beats per minute)

Age	Target Heart Rate (50 –75% of max.)	Average Maximum Heart Rate
20	100–150	200
25	98–146	195
30	95–142	190
35	93–138	185
40	90–135	180
45	88–131	175
50	85–127	170
55	83–123	165
60	80–120	160
65	78–116	155
70	75–113	150

Source: *Exercise and Your Heart: A Guide to Physical Activity.* (1993). National Institutes of Health. National Heart, Lung and Blood Institute.
Note: A few high blood pressure medicines lower the maximum heart rate and thus the target zone rate. If you are taking high blood pressure medications, call your physician to find out if your exercise program needs to be adjusted.

Heart Rate Calculation To determine your heart rate, place the tips of your first two fingers over one of the blood vessels on your neck (carotid arteries) located to the left or right of your Adam's apple. Another convenient pulse spot is the inside of your wrist just below the base of your thumb. Count your pulse for 10 seconds, then multiply by six to give you your heart rate.

EXERCISE SIDE EFFECTS

Exercises For Flexibility, Muscle Tone, And Relaxation

Regular exercise improves balance and coordination and will therefore prevent many of the falls which seem to occur as one ages. This, in addition to adequate bone density, can keep many women from suffering the ill-fated fall which leads to a hip fracture. Although many facilities offer weight training programs, elaborate equipment is not really necessary. Women can lift household objects such as medium-sized or large cans of food, books, or the telephone directory. Light dumbbells can also be purchased in most sporting goods and department stores. For toning and upper body strength, one, two, and three pound weights can be used. Start out gradually with lighter weight objects, and gradually increase both the weight and length of time. Perform lifting activities for at least a half-hour three times a week and involve each muscle group. See Figure 3-9, the "Bone-Saving Fitness Plan" which will contribute to both bone density and strength. Yoga too, contributes to flexibility, induces relaxation, and can be especially effective with sit-ups, push-ups, bending, and stretching.[16]

Exercise has important psychologic effects. Physical activity improves mood, well-being (especially following exercise), and decreases mild anxiety, depression, and stress. There is no denying you will feel better.

Isn't There A Better Way?

Well, you're in luck. Researchers have found that "an active lifestyle does not require a regimented, vigorous exercise program." New physical activity guidelines released jointly by the American College of Sports Medicine and the Centers for Disease Control and Prevention (CDC) specify that individuals should **accumulate** 30 minutes of moderate intense physical activity over most, preferably all, days of the week. The emphasis is on developing activity patterns that can be integrated into daily routines. The 30 minutes can be short bouts such as walking up stairs, taking walks, or doing calisthenics. Gardening, housework, raking leaves, and dancing can contribute to the 30 minutes if done with the same intensity as a brisk walk. For those who perform lower intensity activities, they need to do them longer and more often or both. The experts believe that an increase in fitness will keep people out of nursing homes. The key to all of this is to keep moving regularly, not just in "bouts and spurts"![17,18]

SAFETY

Safety is a big item these days for everyone, but especially for women. When you exercise outdoors, you are placed in a vulnerable position, that is, you may be alone. Use caution when you exercise. Do not run or walk by yourself if you can avoid it. If you do not have a partner, keep the following in mind.

- If alone, run or walk in what you know are safe places; exercise in well-populated, well-lighted places.

- If you must exercise alone, try to let someone know your departure and arrival times.

- Avoid doorways, dense shrubs, or alleys.

- Do not walk or run before dawn or after dark.

- Always be on the lookout for suspicious people or circumstances, for example, an abandoned, parked car.

- If you hear a car or footsteps behind you, turn around and assess the situation.

- Do not wear head phones. As appealing as they may be, they restrict your hearing the approach of a potential attacker or motor vehicle.

- Avoid exercising on busy roadways if possible. If no other alternatives are available, try to avoid peak traffic, run on the shoulder, and face traffic.

- Stay in single file if in a group. Pedestrians usually do not have the right-of-way except in walkways and in intersections.

- Cyclists should obey many of the same rules as the runner or jogger except cyclists should ride with the traffic since they are considered a vehicle with the same rights and responsibilities as an automobile.

- Always be on the defensive. Carry mace, a whistle, or some kind of a siren device.

- Always carry some kind of identification with your name, address, person to contact in an emergency, and any pertinent medical information.

- For women who travel and stay in hotels or motels, the parking lot may be the safest place to jog or walk. Do not attempt out of the way picturesque walking paths. Even in parking lots, watch where you are going. If you must, it is better to run around the entrance to the hotel or motel 100 times than risk the isolated parking lot where danger may lurk between parked cars and vans, especially at dusk and in the early morning daylight hours.

- Check with the hotel concierge regarding safe routes and inform hotel staff of your route and approximate return time. Refer to the resource section for information on the American Running & Fitness Association's "Running Trail Map Network" for a guide to jogging routes in more than 100 cities

EXERCISE MACHINES

Since more and more people have both an interest and access to exercise machines, many questions have been raised regarding the benefits derived from their use. The National Osteoporosis Foundation has developed some useful guidelines, which follow, concerning the purchase or use of these machines and associated benefits.[19]

While exercise machines can provide cardiovascular benefit, improve balance, muscle tone, and overall fitness, they do not provide as much impact as walking briskly up and down hills out-of-doors, jogging, running or other weight-bearing activities described in this book. These machines do provide some degree of weight-bearing exercise as well as some muscular resistance but there has been no research comparing different machines and their impact on bone health.

Since the amount of weight-bearing and impact has an influence on bone density, the greater the amount and force, the greater the benefit. Slow walking delivers less impact than fast walking or jogging. The impact is also related to the body part that takes the impact. For example jogging or walking creates an impact from the foot which is transferred to the leg, hip, and lower spine. The bones of the arm receive no beneficial effect.

Playing tennis improves the bone density only of the arm that hits the ball, and running around the court improves the bone density in the legs, hips and lower spine.

For most people, exercise machines provide too little weight-bearing or impact type exercise to protect current bone health, however they are an excellent alternative in inclement weather and help users remain physically active and fit. They should be an addition or variation to your existing exercise program, not a substitution for it. A varied exercise program is also a more complete program since different muscles and bones are used, thus these machines can be a valuable addition.

The following guidelines, including your own strengths and limitations plus physician recommendation should be considered prior to using or purchasing exercise machines. Before purchasing any machine, you should try it out for 5 to 10 minutes or more and on more than one occasion.

The Treadmill

The treadmill is a machine that allows a person to walk, jog, or run indoors on a cushioned platform. It provides some weight-bearing and impact exercise. Both motorized and non-motorized platforms are available.

What to Look For First, try out several machines. Platforms should have an adequate cushion which absorbs shock and protects joints. They should have safety rails which are high enough so that the user can hold on without bending or leaning forward from the waist, Try the incline and speed controls. Quality treadmills reach 8-12 mph. Walk or run for more than a few minutes and then see how your legs and feet feel the next day or two.

Motorized or Non-motorized A good heavy-duty motorized treadmill is expensive, with the average one costing about $1000. Spending a little more money will often pay off if it ensures a better quality machine. The higher the horsepower, the stronger the machine. Look for machines that have a continuous motor rating of 1.5 horsepower. If given the choice of AC or DC, choose DC since the motors are quieter, offer a wider range of speeds, start slower, and go faster. Choose a control panel with push pads. Built in automatic programs which vary the speed, length and incline often increase the price of the machine, and are not really necessary.

Non-motorized treadmills are less expensive and may or may not have an adjustable incline. Your stride has to push the belt backwards, thus they provide a more strenuous workout.

Motorized treadmills should have emergency stop mechanisms which attach to your clothing causing the machine to stop should you fall or lose your balance.

Elevation Both motorized and non-motorized treadmills come with an incline adjustment that creates a sensation of walking up hill. The ability to change the incline is an important feature since walking or jogging flat on a treadmill is like running slightly downhill.

Belt Size The belt is what you walk or run on, and it is important to get a treadmill with an adequate belt. Belts should be at least 50 inches long and 16 inches wide. Longer, wider belts are safest, with the ideal belt being 18-20 inches wide and 54 inches long.

Handrails A handrail is an important safety feature to be used if you lose your balance. However, leaning on the handrail reduces the amount of weight-bearing effort and throws off your posture. Swing your arms naturally as you do when walking or running. Always land heel first on the belt and keep your head up.

The Ski Machine

A ski machine provides weight-bearing exercise with little or no impact, thus it is easy on the joints of the knee and hip. Some machines allow you to change the incline and adjust the resistance to change the difficulty of the workout.

It has a front upright bar that has a padded bolster against which you lean your abdomen. It has either movable ropes or poles for arm movement and ski-like boards on rollers or foot pads on wheels for leg movement.

Types of Ski Machines There are two types, those with "dependent" skis that are linked, where moving one ski forward pushes the other ski backward.

Those with "independent" skis allow each ski to move individually. The dependent skis force the legs into an awkward stiff shuffle, while independent skis feel more natural but require coordination and practice to master. Although the independent ski machine is more difficult to master, the gait is smoother and has the potential for a more vigorous workout.

The Stair-Climber

Stair-climbers consist of two platforms or pedals that alternately drop under your weight to simulate climbing up stairs or ladder rungs. Steppers may come with handles that are stationary or mobile. Motorized stair-climbers allow the user to change the resistance or effort required for each step, which allows a more intensive workout. While stair-climbers tend to provide less impact and, less jarring to the knees and hip joints, they do strengthen the muscles in the legs, hips, and spine. Stair-climbers provide weight-bearing exercise with more impact than the ski machine, but less impact than the treadmill.

What to Look For Stair-Climbers should be sturdy and not easily tipped over if you lean too far in any direction. When using the stair-climber, feet should remain parallel to the floor. The platforms or pedals should function independently of each other, remain parallel to the ground, and allow the resistance to be adjusted.

The Exercise Bicycle

Exercise bicycles are easy to use because they require the least learning, balance or coordination. The pedals turn a flywheel, fan or both. Resistance can be changed on flywheel models without increasing speed. On fan models, the only way to increase the resistance is to pedal faster. The problem with cycling is that the activity uses fewer muscles than the other machine workouts, and provides no impact, so it is not as good for the bones

What to Look For The seat should feel comfortable and should be adjustable. The height should adjust so that your legs extend almost completely when the pedal is all the way down. Alignment of your knee and ankle is also important.

Considerations Before Making Your Purchase

Prior to purchasing a machine, try it out for at least 5 to 10 minutes. Some stores will allow a trial period in your home which is even better. Regardless of the kind of machine you purchase, it should feel sturdy, move smoothly, be reasonably quiet and allow you to get on and off easily. The machine should also fit your body size comfortably.

EXERCISE AND DISEASE PREVENTION

Exercise makes us look and feel good, but the wonderful effects of exercise go beyond appearance and a general feeling of fitness. Exercise also can improve our health. While performing exercise routines, a sense of strength and agility is noticeable. What we do not notice is the effect exercise has on preventing disease. Being aware of the link between exercise and disease prevention should make a workout program that much more rewarding.

We all know that a healthy lifestyle prevents heart disease, and routine, vigorous, physical activity is a part of any worthwhile health maintenance program. Adequate bone density helps to prevent diseases such as osteoporosis. Weight-bearing and muscle-resistance exercise serves to increase bone density and therefore plays a part in disease prevention. Some evidence, although limited, suggests that exercise may also help prevent other diseases such as cancer. It seems that many of the problems associated with aging cannot be blamed totally on the aging process, but also on a lack of activity which leads to what is known as a sedentary lifestyle.[20,21,22]

The human body has mechanisms that defend against disease constantly. These defense mechanisms involve the immune system. Growing evidence suggests that moderate exercise has a positive effect on the immune system. General and athletic populations alike have found that a certain amount of moderate, regular exercise decreases the chances of getting a cold or flu. A survey conducted by *Runner's World* revealed that more than half of those surveyed said they had fewer colds since they had started running. Severe exertion increased the risk.

Mental fitness and physical fitness cannot be separated. One always affects the other. Because of this connection, it is not surprising to know that physical fitness has been shown to improve mental health.

Exercise and common sense go together. As with most things, moderation is helpful but excess may cause harm. The same is true of exercise. Exercise in moderation will make our bodies feel, look, and work better while severe exertion may expose us to unnecessary risk of injury.

More and more evidence points to the fact that moderate exercise must be a part of the healthy lifestyle we all desire. Exercise helps us to feel good which encourages us to get more out of life. This healthy enthusiasm attracts other people which usually improves our social well-being also. With all of these positive physical, mental, and social benefits, exercise should be a major activity in our lives.

STRESS

Stress seems to be an inevitable part of life. There is absolutely no way to avoid it. The key is to learn to live with it, or better yet, cope with it. Even positive events in our life can be stressful such as marriage, whether it is the first or second; a promotion; or a once-in-a-lifetime experience. Negative events are hard enough, but they are made worse when our support systems are limited or lacking. Poor coping skills also affect the amount of stress an event can cause.

Coping With Stress

We all know the best way to eliminate stress is to avoid whatever causes it, but how realistic is this? Women today have very unrealistic expectations of themselves. These expectations can intensify an already stressful situation. Many women try to be "everything to everybody." Elimination of some stressful factors might be possible if time is taken to examine what is at stake. Change what you can; and when you cannot change the situation, learn to cope or live it. Limit the number of stressful situations if that is possible.

Although there are a number of resources available, only a few very basic suggestions will be offered here. Professional help should be investigated for those who feel more help is needed or if things seem to be out of control.

Healthy Life Style Probably the best way to be successful in coping with stressful situations is through a healthy lifestyle which includes none other than what you have read so far—balanced diet, adequate sleep, and exercise. Physical activity is probably one of the best kinds of stress prevention around. Approximately 90 minutes after a vigorous bout of exercise, a certain calm or tranquility envelops the body. Regular exercisers know the feeling, and are aware of its lasting effects throughout the day. The mental attitude becomes more positive and a person is better able to cope with stress. Physical exercise actually contributes to a state of well-being, because the body feels right (and conversely, feels wrong without exercise). Exercise enables us to have positive feelings about our-selves and this positive feeling is noticed by others.[23] Even a novice will be able to reap the psychological benefits of exer-cise. Physical activity makes us feel healthy, much like when we eat a well-balanced diet. All of this not only prevents us from becoming easily stressed, but it also equips us to better deal with stress when we cannot avoid it.

Thus, a combination of a good diet, adequate sleep, and physical activity allows us to feel refreshed and in better con-trol of our lives which in turn allows us to control other sit-uations that confront us regularly. It really sounds too simple, doesn't it? But it does work if you are conscientious about eating the right kind of diet described in this book, getting adequate amounts of sleep, and exercising regularly! And you must live on a regular routine or schedule. The human body was designed to live in harmony with all of its parts. If you want to be able to cope with life and enjoy it to its fullest, a daily routine is a must!

Relaxation Having said all of this, there are times when we may need a bit of help, and this does not mean the kind of help provided through the use of alcohol or drugs. These are only temporary measures, may be habit forming, and lead nowhere. The missing part of all of this is learning to relax.

- The easiest advice you have often heard is "take a deep breath." Do just that! Take a deep breath, hold it for 5 seconds, and...breathe out. Let your body go loose as you breathe out. Continue to do this as long as you can depending upon the circumstances. Then, slowly resume your normal breathing pattern. You will be surprised at how effective it can be, and it can be done most any place and any time.

- You may also use the breathing exercise to set the stage for a more intense relaxation exercise. An example of one can be found in Appendix B. It will require some practice and concentration to learn how to do it, there-fore, do not be discouraged the first few times you try it.

Exercise

Although many benefits of exercise as a preventive measure have been described, physical activity as a treatment measure in stress management has not.

Fight Or Flight Let us examine three stressful situations all of which have the same end result.

1. A working woman strives to achieve a promotion. Having been selected as a finalist to make a special presentation before the entire department, she prepares at great length. Yet one person in the group is out to jeopardize her chances to the point of humiliation, and manages to "do her in."

2. A woman works long and hard hours to arrange the perfect fund raiser. During the final preparations, disaster occurs, people have not followed through on their responsibilities, and everything seems to be falling apart. Everyone is blaming her.

3. A woman finds out her best friend just ran away with her husband.

Can you feel the tension? This directionless, explosive energy is often referred to as "the fight or flight" response. This stress response in us was intended to end in physical activity. The body prepares by

- pouring out sugar and fat into the system to feed the muscles and the brain,

- dilating the pupils for better visual acuity, and

- increasing heart and respiration rates to pump blood and oxygen to active muscles and stimulate control centers in the brain.

This is not a time to sit, but to **move**, to relieve the body of the negative forces of stress on the system. Now is the time for some vigorous activity such as swimming, running, dancing, biking, a brisk walk, a few quick trips up and down a set of stairs (that is, of course if you are physically fit enough to do so) to use up the stress products that would normally play a part in causing heart or stomach problems.[23]

Some of you may respond with "circumstances just won't allow me to do that." The better question is "How can I afford not to take the time to release the energy in a healthy, productive manner?" If you feel it may do you some good, you will no doubt find the "release valve" that works. Or better yet, if you take care of yourself and engage in a vigorous exercise routine, you will be in a better position to deal with these stressors.

COMMITMENT

Diet and exercise are joint partners that work together to make us physically and mentally sound not just for today, but for the future that awaits us. Commitment to a healthy lifestyle should begin in the teenage years, but any day is a good day to start.

Women And Research

Each preceding chapter has touched on research issues in some way. Research has given us the answers to what we know about women's health today, and it will be the source of tomorrow's answers. But a great deal of controversy exists concerning research and women. During the last few years, it has been found that women have been neglected in the research arena. Questions have been raised regarding whether enough research monies have been allocated to women's health issues, whether women are adequately represented in clinical trials, and whether treatment success differs between men and women.[1] Any woman experiencing a change in her body like menopause wants clear, accurate answers to her questions. Conflicting information makes health choices that much more difficult. Understanding the research situation will provide a picture of why confusing information exists, and will also provide a basis for being able to read about new information with a critical eye. Just as women have had to fight for equal rights in the board room, so must they protect themselves in the health arena.

RESEARCH IN A "NUTSHELL"

To better understand the research process, a few basic facts must be understood.

Epidemiology

Medical science has its own branch of research that deals with the interrelationships of (in this case) the human body or host, disease causing agents, and the environment in which both exist. This branch is called epidemiology. Epidemiology determines how a host, an agent, and their environment work together to cause disease. An example of an epidemiologic study might involve postmenopausal females (the host) and osteoporosis (a disease experienced by postmenopausal females) plus the addition of prescribed hormones to determine their effect on both the disease and the host.

Observational Versus Clinical Studies Epidemiologic studies are often described as either observational or clinical studies or trials. Knowing the difference between the two helps a person to determine how the study was carried out. In observational trials, the epidemiologist merely observes a group; no interaction takes place. Clinical studies, on the other hand, are planned experiments where the researcher manipulates the situation. Usually in clinical trials, one group of test subjects may receive treatment while others do not. The effects of both methods are then compared.

Test Populations

For a test or experiment to have meaning, the number of subjects studied must be large, and the individual characteristics of the subjects selected for study should not unfairly influence the results.

Population Size To assess the health effects of studies appropriately, the subject population must be large enough to detect changes produced from treatment and generate enough data to create statistics that have meaning. The following is an example of what can happen if the test group is too small. If 10 women are studied and one develops cancer, then statistically 1 in 10 women will develop cancer. But say 1000 women were tested and only one develops cancer, the chance of getting cancer is now 1 in 1000. For any test, the sample size must be large enough to produce realistic data. Observational studies, by their very design, usually have larger sample sizes than clinical studies.

Random Selection The example just used helps demonstrate the idea of random selection. What if the 1000 women tested all live on a beautiful, smog-free tropical island and eat wild berries and plants all day. Would you question the results? Of course, you would. This experiment would have little meaning to a woman who breathes industrial smoke, eats fast food, and balances home and work. The practice of choosing subjects to ensure fair results is termed "random selection." The purpose of the random selection process is to equalize other causes of treatment or nontreatment results across groups. An example of "random selection" might be taking a population of 500 women who are on HRT and choosing 200 of them by using a method that will guarantee that each of the 500 has an equal chance of being included in the study group of 200. A comparison group, not on treatment, is selected using the same method. Both observational and clinical studies can utilize random selection to decrease the chance of bias being introduced into a study.

Although helpful, the random selection process is not perfect. Researchers may admit test subjects into a study only to find out later that they have certain lifestyles or habits that may bias the study. A bias that is discovered after the study begins can be statistically removed, meaning that at the end of the experiment, the results from the subjects creating the bias are removed from the data.

Ethics

Tests cannot be performed anytime, anywhere, or anyway. Very strict rules govern the research process. If ethical considerations did not exist, testing would be an easy process. Consider for the moment that a researcher wants to study the effects of estrogen on women who have had a hysterectomy. This researcher cannot solicit subjects for the test and then perform a hysterectomy on each. That obviously, would be unethical. The only path open to this scientist would be to find women who have already had hysterectomies and ask for their cooperation. Time may be lost, but subject rights are maintained.

Funding

Research costs money. Many worthwhile test ideas exist, but who gets the funding is tightly controlled by government and private organizations. Women should know if an equal share of the research monies are being devoted to their concerns.

Time

The human body usually experiences change slowly; therefore, tests performed on the human body usually take time. This slow process can be very frustrating and discouraging, because people need answers now. Yet testing should be allowed sufficient time in order to detect effects that may occur only after relatively long treatment. We know smoking does not cause long-term lung problems after one cigarette; it takes time before the harmful effects can cause irreversible damage. So, too, with diseases like osteoporosis, bone density decreases over time, and time is needed for treatment to stop the effects of osteoporosis. Human tests can last anywhere from a few days, to years, to decades and beyond. Many of the tests involving menopause and other women's health issues are long range tests. This is precisely why women need to concern themselves with research issues. Starting these tests now will assure answers in the future.

Methodology

Researchers can only utilize what is available to them. For example, Premarin, a widely prescribed estrogen, may appear in many studies because of the length of time it has been available in the United States. Other forms of estrogen have not been tested because researchers do not have access to them. Although some forms of estrogen are used in Europe, they have not been approved for use in the United States. If not approved, researchers cannot always use them in their tests, so information on these drugs is lacking. Even though new forms of estrogen administration are now accepted, such as the transdermal skin patch, time is needed to perform the studies and gather the results.

Validity

First time study results may generate a lot of excitement, but test data is only to be believed when it can be duplicated again and again in other tests.

WHERE DO WE STAND?

The question of women's issues being neglected by research has not been ignored. In the late 1980s, an inventory of various types of funded research by the National Institutes of Health (NIH) was conducted. The study showed that 13% of NIH research was in the area of women's health, 10% centered on men's health issues, and the rest dealt with areas that affect both men and women. This inventory and its results did not stop the controversy, because it did not touch on the real problems.

THE PROBLEMS

Focus was not directed toward the 77% of research dealing with men and women. The NIH inventory never determined the number of female test subjects in the 77% population.[1] An alarming number of medical studies have shown an inadequate number of female subjects, if not a complete lack of women in studies.

Why should women be left out of research? The three reasons usually given are 1) women complicate research results because of their hormonal fluctuations, 2) women could cause legal and ethical problems if they became pregnant during the studies, and 3) women's health issues are secondary to men's.[2]

Because of this type of research practice, the reactions of men to tests have been made the standard. This means that results of studies conducted on men are automatically applied to women. The assumption must be that no differences exist between men and women. How strange it is that researchers recognize differences between the sexes during the experimental phase by neglecting to use women as test subjects, but seem to deny these differences when it comes to the test results.

A test performed in the 1970s on the protective effects of estrogen against heart attack followed this thinking. All test subjects were men and the results showed that estrogen provided no benefit in the prevention of heart attacks. Later estrogen studies on women found estrogen to be quite beneficial.

This book has already discussed the fact that women differ in physiological makeup from men, and that their risk for heart attack and stroke compared to men of the same age is different. These few examples alone should persuade researchers that men's reactions to treatments cannot be held as the standard for women.

ACTION

The NIH inventory did not go unchallenged. In 1989, the Congressional Caucus for Women's Issues insisted on change. The Office of Research on Women's Health was created in 1990 to make certain that women and women's health problems were included in NIH funded studies.

Women's Health Initiative
Probably the greatest result has come in the form of the "Women's Health Initiative." This $625 million, 14 year project, the largest of its kind, will study disease in women as they age. Nearly 150,000 women will take part in this study at some 45 clinical centers across the United States.

This Initiative has two important goals. The first is to decrease the prevalence of cardiovascular disease, cancer (especially breast cancer), and osteoporosis among women. The outcome should provide health care providers with recommendations on diet, hormone replacement therapy, diet supplements, and exercise to be used by women of all ethnic groups and socioeconomic classes. The second, related goal will focus on older women and evaluate methods for motivating these older women to adopt health-enhancing behaviors.[2] Research on the middle years of a woman's life is definitely a high priority item in the Office of Research on Women's Health.

HISTORICAL STUDIES

Of the studies that have been performed, some studies have occurred which have shaped our thoughts on women's health today. These studies are worth mention.

The Baltimore Longitudinal Study Of Aging

The Baltimore Longitudinal Study of Aging (BLSA) funded by the National Institute on Aging of the National Institutes of Health began in 1958. The major focus was to investigate normal aging. Initial findings have shown that prior to menopause, women have a lower incidence of heart disease and high blood pressure. This study is also important in demonstrating that the diagnosis of heart disease differs between men and women.

The Framingham Study

The Framingham Study was funded by the National Heart, Lung, and Blood Institute of NIH in 1948. The plan was to identify the relationship between sex, heredity, and environment on atherosclerotic and hypertensive (high blood pressure) heart disease. Environmental factors included education, smoking, occupation, and physical activity. Several menopause-related findings were discovered.

1) Smokers experienced menopause approximately a year earlier than nonsmokers.
2) Cardiovascular disease increased with menopause, as did the severity of the disease.
3) Elevated hemoglobin (oxygen carrying capacity of the blood) and serum cholesterol levels were found in postmenopausal women when compared to premenopausal women.

Offspring of the participants of the original Framingham study have also been studied. This study involved postmenopausal estrogen users and blood cholesterol levels. The results showed that estrogen users had higher levels of good cholesterol (HDL) and lower levels of bad cholesterol (LDL) than nonusers. Unfortunately, neither study investigated the effect of progesterone on cardiovascular disease.

The Healthy Women Study

In 1983, another menopause transition study known as the Healthy Women Study was supported by the National Heart, Lung, and Blood Institute of NIH. This five-year study related behavioral and biological characteristics to disease, especially cardiovascular disease. Subjects with any existing disease condition were removed from the study. Although no effect was found on blood pressure, glucose metabolism, and caloric expenditure or consumption during the menopause transition period, there was a decline in HDL and an increase in LDL. Furthermore, the estrogen (with or without progesterone) users had improved lipoprotein and cholesterol levels, which put them at decreased risk for cardiovascular disease.[1]

The Leisure World Study

Female residents of a retirement community in southern California participated in the Leisure World Study which began in 1981. The participants were approximately 73 years of age, most were White, well educated, and comfortable financially. Mortality and estrogen use were compared. The use of estrogen postmenopausally was associated with a 20% reduction in mortality from all causes. This reduction did not depend on the dosage of estrogen used, but was greatest with long durations of use. Deaths related to heart disease and stroke also decreased. Unfortunately, few women took progestins or parenteral (injectable) estrogens, so the effect of those hormones on mortality could not be determined.[3,4]

The Nurses Health Study

The Nurses Health Study, cited earlier, and funded by various institutes of NIH, has been charting the medical history of approximately 120,000 female nurses since 1976. The main objective of the study was to determine the relationships among lifestyle and environmental components. A mailed questionnaire asked participants about previous cardiovascular disease, menopause, diabetes, high blood pressure, high cholesterol levels, and parental heart attacks. The nurses revealed information on height, weight, smoking, the use of postmenopausal hormones, and the use of oral contraceptives. Every two years, the participants fill out a follow-up questionnaire. A dietary questionnaire was added in 1980.

Results already show a decreased risk for heart disease in current estrogen users and a 30% increased risk of breast cancer among women who consumed between three and nine drinks of alcohol per week.[1] The latest results on breast cancer risk have shown an increased incidence in long time estrogen users suggesting the need for a careful assessment between risks and benefits for these women. However final results are still inconclusive because of shortcomings in the methodology and population bias.[5,6] This study is also taking a look at progesterone use. Estrogen therapy with progesterone has shown a decreased risk of uterine cancer while estrogen therapy alone has indicated a reduced risk of ovarian cancer.

The Postmenopausal Estrogen/Progestin Interventions Trials

Funded by many Institutes at NIH, the Postmenopausal Estrogen/Progestin Interventions Trials (PEPI) collected information on the cardiovascular effects of estrogen and several different combinations of estrogen and progestin. Individuals on estrogen alone or in combination with progestin showed improved lipoprotein or lipid levels and lower clotting factor levels (both of which are responsible for cardiovascular problems). Bone density improved in women on estrogen alone and in those on the combined estrogen and progestin regimen.[7]

PEPI had many critics; the opposition felt PEPI was too short to provide solid answers to the effect of HRT on heart disease, stroke, and osteoporosis. Differences in types of estrogen administration methods could not be studied since oral estrogen alone was used. Nevertheless, PEPI was a controlled clinical trial, and therefore more reliable than the observational studies, and in some cases has eliminated some of the myths and uncertainties associated with the use of HRT.[8,9]

The Women's Health Study

The Women's Health Study involving 40,000 healthy post-menopausal females with no history of cancer or heart disease began in 1992 to investigate the relationship of beta carotene, aspirin, and vitamin E to cancer (lung, breast, and colon) and cardiovascular disease. The results will compliment data currently being gathered on the effects of beta carotene in men.

The National Institutes of Health are funding this study to be conducted by Harvard Medical School and Brigham and Women's Hospital in Boston, Massachusetts.

Although the focus of the Women's Health Study is on heart disease and cancer risk factors, other issues about breast implants, tissue disorders, breast cancer, and the relationship of aspirin to migraine headache prevention are involved.[10,11]

The Heart And Estrogen/Progesterone Replacement Study

The final study to be reviewed is "HERS," Heart and Estrogen/Progesterone Replacement Study. This five-year study will examine postmenopausal women with documented heart disease and with an intact uterus. One half of the women will be put on hormone therapy and the other half on placebos.

DRUG RESEARCH AND WOMEN

The fact that individuals react differently to the same medication is pretty obvious to most people. Penicillin is a good example of how one person can take a medication and experience relief while another will take it and develop an allergic reaction. Researchers are very aware of personal reactions to medications. It is known that drug response in the body can be affected by age, body size, gender, body fat content, pre-existing illness, and medications taken at the same time. If individuals can be so diverse, doesn't it make sense that men and women might have different responses? Body fat, body composition, and hormones are thought to be major factors which are responsible for different drug responses between men and women. Because of inadequate information about gender differences, the Food and Drug Administration (FDA) in 1993 developed steps to ensure that new drugs are appropriately evaluated in women. These new guidelines require that a sufficient number of women of all ages be enrolled in new drug studies. The studies will note how much drug is retained in the body over time and how the body responds to different dosages. The FDA also changed a policy that had previously excluded women of "childbearing potential" from the early phases of clinical drug trials. Related to this change, the new guidelines call for appropriate measures for minimizing the risk of fetal exposure.[12]

FILLING THE RESEARCH GAPS

The tide is changing as more research begins to focus specifically on women's health topics, but vigilance must be maintained to prevent a shift back to earlier practices. Many questions are left without answers, but as long as research continues the answers will come.

Appendix A

A Sample Walking Program*

	Warm up	Target zone exercising	Cool down	Total time
Week 1				
Session A	Walk 5 min.	Then walk briskly 5 min.	Then walk more slowly 5 min.	15 min.
Session B	Repeat above pattern			
Session C	Repeat above pattern			

Continue with at least three exercise sessions during each week of the program.

Week 2	Walk 5 min.	Walk briskly 7 min.	Walk 5 min.	17 min.
Week 3	Walk 5 min.	Walk briskly 9 min.	Walk 5 min.	19 min.
Week 4	Walk 5 min.	Walk briskly 11 min.	Walk 5 min.	21 min.
Week 5	Walk 5 min.	Walk briskly 13 min.	Walk 5 min.	23 min.
Week 6	Walk 5 min.	Walk briskly 15 min.	Walk 5 min.	25 min.
Week 7	Walk 5 min.	Walk briskly 18 min.	Walk 5 min.	28 min.
Week 8	Walk 5 min.	Walk briskly 20 min.	Walk 5 min.	30 min.
Week 9	Walk 5 min.	Walk briskly 23 min.	Walk 5 min.	33 min.
Week 10	Walk 5 min.	Walk briskly 26 min.	Walk 5 min.	36 min.
Week 11	Walk 5 min.	Walk briskly 28 min.	Walk 5 min.	38 min.
Week 12	Walk 5 min.	Walk briskly 30 min.	Walk 5 min.	40 min.

Week 13 on:

Check your pulse periodically to see if you are exercising within your target zone. As you become more fit, try exercising within the upper range of your target zone. Gradually increase your brisk walking time to 30 to 60 minutes, three or four times a week. Remember that your goal is to get the benefits you are seeking and enjoy your activity.

Source: A Sample Walking Program. (1993). *Exercise and Your Heart: A Guide to Physical Activity.* NATIONAL INSTITUTES OF HEALTH. National Heart, Lung and Blood Institute. American Heart Association.

A Sample Jogging Program*

Note: If you are over 40 and have not been active, you should not begin with a program as strenuous as jogging. Begin with the walking program instead. After completing the walking program, you can start with week 3 of the jogging program.

	Warm up	Target zone exercising	Cool down	Total time
Week 1				
Session A	Walk 5 min., then stretch and limber up	Then walk 10 min. Try not to stop	Then walk slowly 3 min. and stretch 2 min.	20 min.
Session B	Repeat above pattern			
Session C	Repeat above pattern			

Continue with at least three exercise sessions during each week of the program.

	Warm up	Target zone exercising	Cool down	Total time
Week 2	Walk 5 min., then stretch and limber up	Walk 5 min., jog 1 min., walk 5 min., jog 1 min.	Walk 3 min., stretch 2 min.	22 min.
Week 3	Walk 5 min., then stretch and limber up	Walk 5 min., jog 3 min., walk 5 min., jog 3 min.	Walk 3 min., stretch 2 min.	26 min.
Week 4	Walk 5 min., then stretch and limber up	Walk 4 min., jog 5 min., walk 4 min., jog 5 min.	Walk 3 min., stretch 2 min.	28 min.
Week 5	Walk 5 min., then stretch and limber up	Walk 4 min., jog 5 min., walk 4 min., jog 5 min.	Walk 3 min., stretch 2 min.	28 min.
Week 6	Walk 5 min., then stretch and limber up	Walk 4 min., jog 6 min., walk 4 min., jog 6 min.	Walk 3 min., stretch 2 min.	30 min.
Week 7	Walk 5 min., then stretch and limber up	Walk 4 min., jog 7 min., walk 4 min., jog 7 min.	Walk 3 min., stretch 2 min.	32 min.
Week 8	Walk 5 min., then stretch and limber up	Walk 4 min., jog 8 min., walk 4 min., jog 8 min.	Walk 3 min., stretch 2 min.	34 min.

Week 9	Walk 5 min., then stretch and limber up	Walk 4 min., jog 9 min., walk 4 min., jog 9 min.	Walk 3 min., stretch 2 min.	36 min.
Week 10	Walk 5 min., then stretch and limber up	Walk 4 min., jog 13 min.	Walk 3 min., stretch 2 min.	27 min.
Week 11	Walk 5 min., then stretch and limber up	Walk 4 min., jog 15 min.	Walk 3 min., stretch 2 min.	29 min.
Week 12	Walk 5 min., then stretch and limber up	Walk 4 min., jog 17 min.	Walk 3 min., stretch 2 min.	31 min.
Week 13	Walk 5 min., then stretch and limber up	Walk 2 min., jog slowly 2 min., jog 17 min.	Walk 3 min., stretch 2 min.	31 min.
Week 14	Walk 5 min., then stretch and limber up	Walk 1 min., jog slowly 3 min., jog 17 min.	Walk 3 min., stretch 2 min.	31 min.
Week 15	Walk 5 min., then stretch and limber up	jog slowly 3 min., jog 17 min.	Walk 3 min., stretch 2 min.	30 min.

Week 16 on:

Check your pulse periodically to see if you are exercising within your target zone. As you become more fit, try exercising within the upper range of your target zone. Gradually increase your jogging time from 20 to 30 minutes (or more, up to 60 minutes), three or four times a week. Your goal is to get the benefits you are seeking and enjoy your activity.

Source: A Sample Jogging Program. (1993). *Exercise and Your Heart: A Guide to Physical Activity.* NATIONAL INSTITUTES OF HEALTH. National Heart, Lung and Blood Institute. American Heart Association.

*The exercise patterns for both of the sample programs are suggested guidelines. Listen to your body and build up less quickly, if needed.

Appendix B
Putting it All Together

The 8-Minute Relaxation Plan

Minute 1 In a quiet room and in a comfortable chair assume a restful position and a quiet, passive attitude. Take four deep breaths. Make each one deeper than the one before: Hold the first inhalation for 4 seconds, the second one for 5 seconds, the third one for 6 seconds, and the fourth one for 7 seconds. Pull the tension from all parts of your body into your lungs and exhale it with each expiration. Feel more relaxed with each breath.

Minute 2 Count backward from 10 to 0. Breathe naturally, and with each exhalation count one number and feel more and more relaxed as you approach 0. With each count you descend a relaxation stairway and become more deeply relaxed until you are totally relaxed at 0.

Minutes 3-7 Now, use your imagination and go to a relaxation place that you have either been to or can imagine, one which is peaceful and has a calming, pleasant effect. Stay there for four minutes. Try to vividly, but passively, recall the feeling of that place and time that were very relaxing.

Minute 8 Bring your attention back to yourself. Count from 0 to 10. Energize your body. Feel the energy, vitality, and health flow through your system. Feel alert and eager to resume your activities. Open your eyes.

Note: From *Controlling Stress and Tension: A Holistic Approach* (p.218), by D. A. Girdano and G. S. Everly, 1979, Englewood Cliffs, NJ: Prentice-Hall, Inc. Copyright 1995 by Allyn and Bacon. Adapted by permission.

Glossary

Amenorrhea—absence or abnormal stoppage of the menses.

Androgen/androgenic—any substance, e.g., androsterone and testosterone, that stimulates male characteristics.

Angina—a disease marked by brief attacks of chest pain.

Angiogram—a picture of a blood vessel filled with a contrasting material.

Areola—the area of dark-colored skin that surrounds the nipple.

Arthralgia—pain in a joint; experienced by some women during the climacteric.

Aspiration—removal of fluid from a lump with a needle.

Atherosclerosis—a type of "hardening of the arteries" in which cholesterol, fat and other blood components build up on the inner lining of the arteries.

Atrophy—a wasting away; a decrease in the size of a cell, tissue, organ or body part.

Atypical hyperplasia of breast—a benign (noncancerous) condition in which breast tissue has certain abnormal features.

Axilla—the underarm.

Benign—not cancerous; does not invade nearby tissue or spread to other parts of the body.

Biopsy—the removal of a sample of tissue, which is then examined under a microscope to check for cancer cells.

Breakthrough bleeding—any visible unexpected vaginal bleeding.

Cancer—a term for more than 100 diseases in which abnormal cells divide without control. Cancer cells can spread through the bloodstream and lymphatic system to other parts of the body.

Carbohydrate—one of the three nutrients that supply calories to the body. Carbohydrates provide 4 calories per gram—the same number as pure protein and less than half the calories of fat. There are two basic kinds of carbohydrate—simple (sugars) and complex (starches and fiber).

Carcinoma—cancer that begins in the lining or covering of an organ.

Carcinoma in situ—cancer that involves only the tissue in which it began; it has not spread to other tissues.

Cardiovascular disease—diseases pertaining to the heart and blood vessels.

Chemotherapy—treatment with anticancer drugs.

Cholesterol—a soft waxy substance; it is made in sufficient quantity by the body for normal body function, including the manufacture of hormones, bile acid, and vitamin D. It is present in all parts of the body, including the nervous system, muscle, skin, liver, intestines, heart, etc.

Cholesterol (blood)—cholesterol that is manufactured in the liver and absorbed from the food you eat and is carried in the blood for use by all parts of the body. A high level of blood cholesterol leads to atherosclerosis and coronary heart disease.

Cholesterol (dietary)—cholesterol that is in the foods you eat; is found only in foods of animal origin, not foods of plant origin. Dietary cholesterol like saturated fat tends to raise blood cholesterol, which increases the risk for heart disease.

Climacteric—the years leading up to and following the last menstrual period. May frequently be called the perimenopause.

Clinical trials—research studies that involve patients.

Coronary heart disease—heart ailment caused by narrowing of the coronary arteries (arteries that supply oxygen and nutrients directly to the heart muscle).

Corpus luteum—yellow mass in the ovary formed by an ovarian follicle that has matured and discharged its ovum.

Cyst—a closed sac or capsule filled with fluid.

DUB—dysfunctional uterine bleeding; excessive and/or unpredictable bleeding from the uterus, frequently occurs in the few years before menopause; not due to any abnormality.

Dyspareunia—difficult or painful sexual intercourse.

Dysuria—painful or difficult urination.

Endogenous—produced within or caused by factors within the organism.

Endometrium—the tissues lining the uterus (womb).

Epidemiology—study of the relationships of various factors which affect the frequency and distribution of diseases in the human community.

Etiology—the science of dealing with causes of disease.

Exogenous estrogen—estrogen that is not produced by the body but is provided by other means such as tablets, creams, skin patches.

Fat—one of the three nutrients that supply calories to the body; fat provides 9 calories per gram, more than twice the number provided by carbohydrate or protein; small amounts of fat are necessary for normal body function.

Fat (total)—sum of saturated, monounsaturated and polyunsaturated fats in food.

Fat (saturated)—a type of fat found in greatest amounts in foods from animals such as meat, poultry, and whole-milk dairy products like cream, milk, ice cream, and cheese.

Fat (unsaturated)—a type of fat that is usually liquid at refrigerator temperature; monounsaturated fat and polyunsaturated fat are two kinds of unsaturated fat.

Fat (monounsaturated)—a slightly unsaturated fat that is found in greatest amounts in foods from plants, including olive and canola oil; helps reduce blood cholesterol.

Fat (polyunsaturated)—a highly unsaturated fat that is found in greatest amounts in foods from plants, including safflower, sunflower, corn, and soybean oils; helps reduce blood cholesterol.

Fat (omega-3 fatty acid (fish oil)—a type of polyunsaturated fat found in seafood and found in greatest amounts in fatty fish; seafood is lower in saturated fat than meat.

FSH—follicle-stimulating hormone; stimulates development of sacs that hold the eggs.

Gram (g)—a unit of weight; there are about 28 g in 1 ounce; dietary fat, protein, and carbohydrate are measured in grams.

GnRH—gonadotropin-releasing hormone; stimulates the release of FSH and LH.

Hormones—chemicals produced by glands in the body; hormones control the actions of certain cells or organs.

Hydrogenation—a chemical process that changes liquid vegetable oils (unsaturated fat) into a more solid saturated fat; this process improves the shelf life of the product—but increases the saturated fat content.

Hypermenorrhea—excessive menstrual bleeding, but occurring at regular intervals and being of usual duration.

Hyperplasia—abnormal increase in the number of normal cells in normal arrangement in an organ or tissue, which increases its size.

Hypomenorrhea—diminution of menstrual flow or duration.

Hysterectomy—surgical removal of the uterus (womb).

Leiomyoma—also known as a fibroid; a noncancerous growth in the uterus that occurs before menopause.

LH—luteinizing hormone; stimulates the release of the egg from the sac.

Lipoproteins—protein-coated packages that carry fat and cholesterol through the blood; classified according to their density.

Lipoproteins (high-density)—contain a small amount of cholesterol and carry cholesterol away from body cells and tissues to the liver for elimination from the body.

Lipoproteins (low-density)—contain the largest amount of cholesterol in the blood; responsible for depositing cholesterol in the artery walls.

Lumpectomy—surgery to remove only the cancerous breast lump; usually followed by radiation therapy.

Lymph—the almost colorless fluid that travels through the lymphatic system and carries cells that help fight infection and disease.

Lymph nodes—small bean-shaped organs located along the channels of the lymphatic system; bacteria or cancer cells that enter the lymphatic system may be found in the nodes; also called lymph glands.

Malignant—cancerous; can spread to other parts of the body.

Mammogram—x-ray of the breast.

Mastectomy—surgery to remove the breast.

Menorrhagia—heavy menstrual bleeding and excessively long periods.

Menses—the monthly flow of blood from the female genital tract.

Menstrual cycle—the hormone changes that lead up to a woman having a period; for most women, one cycle takes 28 days.

Metastasis—the spread of cancer from one part of the body to another.

Milligram (mg)—a unit of weight equal to one-thousandth of a gram; there are about 28,350 mg in 1 ounce; dietary cholesterol is measured in milligrams.

Milligrams/deciliter (mg/dl)—a way of expressing concentration: in blood cholesterol measurements, the weight of cholesterol (in milligrams) in a deciliter of blood; a deciliter is about one-tenth of a quart.

Morbidity—the condition of being sick; the sick rate; the ratio of sick to well persons in a community.

Mortality—ratio of actual deaths to expected deaths.

Nulliparity—the state of being a woman who has never borne a live child.

Observational studies—an epidemiologic study in which there is no artificial manipulation of the study factor.

Oligomenorrhea—infrequent menstruation with diminished flow.

Oophorectomy—surgical removal of the ovaries.

Opposed estrogen—estrogen that is used in conjunction with progestin.

Paresthesia—sensation of tingling, prickling or creeping of the skin; experienced by some women during the climacteric.

Peripheral conversion—conversion of estrogen outside of the liver, in the outer tissues.

Platelets—any of the disk-shaped structures in the blood, chiefly known for their role in blood coagulation.

Protein—one of the three nutrients that supply calories to the body; protein provides 4 calories per gram, which is less than half the calories of fat.

Randomized trials—an epidemiologic experiment in which subjects are randomly allocated into groups, the "study" and "control" groups, to receive or not to receive an experimental preventive or therapeutic procedure, for example, a drug.

Selection bias—a distortion in the effect resulting from the manner in which subjects are selected for a study population.

Transdermal—through the skin.

Tumor—an abnormal mass of tissue.

Unopposed estrogen—estrogen used alone.

Urethra—a tube through which urine is discharged from the bladder to the exterior of the body.

Uterus—the hollow muscular organ in the female in which the fertilized ovum (egg) normally becomes embedded and in which the developing embryo and fetus are nourished. Its cavity opens into the vagina below.

Vagina—the canal in the female, from the vulva to the cervix of the uterus, that receives the penis in sexual intercourse, and is the birth canal.

Vaginal atrophy—the wasting or diminution in size of the vagina.

Withdrawal bleeding—"planned" bleeding that occurs during the hormone-free period of a cycle or after progestin has been added to a continuous cycle.

Resources

A select number of resources are listed which will enhance the information provided in this book.

Agency for Health Care Policy and Research
    Publications Clearinghouse
    P.O. Box 8547
    Silver Spring, MD 20907-8547
    (800) 358-9295

    Guidelines on health issues

Alliance for Aging Research
    2021 K Street, NW, Suite 305
    Washington, DC 20006
    (202) 293-2856

American Cancer Society
    1599 Clifton Road, N.E.
    Atlanta, GA 30329
    (800) ACS-2345

    Local chapter may also be contacted for information on prevention, detection, diagnosis and treatment for all types of cancers. All publications and services are free.

American Diabetes Association
    1600 Duke Street
    Alexandria, VA 22314
    (800) 232-3472; (703) 549-1500

    Contact the local chapters or the national office. Offers patient and family education activities such as educational meetings, weekend retreats, counseling and discussion, self-help, and support groups. There are membership fees and costs for some publications.

American Dietetic Association
216 W. Jackson Blvd, Suite 800
Chicago, IL 60606
(312) 899-0040;
(800) 366-1655 (Consumer Nutrition Hotline)

Provides clear and objective nutrition information to callers who are concerned about eating habits, lifestyle choices, and health. Recorded messages in English and Spanish are available Monday through Friday 8:00 am to 8:00 pm central time. Offers cookbooks and other materials for consumers designed to educate about food and nutrition.

American Heart Association (AHA)
National Center
7272 Greenville Ave
Dallas, TX 75231
(214) 373-6300; (800) AHA USA1

Local chapter may also be contacted for information on prevention and treatment of heart disease in women. Special publications on heart disease in women may be available.

American Lung Association (ALA)
1740 Broadway
New York, NY 10019
(212) 315-8700

Local affiliates conduct smoking cessation programs and offer a catalog of publications, including many on smoking. Contact your local affiliate or write to the above address. Some fees may apply.

American Running & Fitness Association
Dept BHG
9310 Old Georgetown Road
Bethesda, MD 20814
1-800 776 ARFA

Running Trail Maps for a variety of cities

Consumer Information Center (CIC)
Pueblo, CO 81009
(719) 948-3334

Consumer Information Catalog from CIC lists over 200 free or low-cost booklets on consumer topics. Many are health-related and include booklets on nutrition, foods, exercise, women's health, and smoking. Write for a free copy.

DEPRESSION Awareness, Recognition, and Treatment Program
National Institute of Mental Health
D/ART Public Inquiries
5600 Fishers Lane
Room 7C-02
Rockville, MD 20857
301) 443-4513

Food and Drug Administration (FDA)
MQSA Consumer Inquiries
1350 Piccard
(HFZ-240)
Rockville, MD 20850
(301) 443-3170

General information on breast cancer and mammography

Food and Drug Administration (FDA)
Office of Consumer Affairs, HFE-88
5600 Fishers Lane
Rockville, MD 20857
(301) 443-3170

Offers publication on topics such as general drug information, medical devices, and food-related subjects. FDA also publishes a monthly journal, FDA Consumer, which reports on recent developments in the regulation of foods, drugs, and cosmetics.

Food and Drug Administration
Consumer Affairs and Information
5600 Fishers Lane, HFC-110
Rockville, MD 20857
(301) 443-3170

To get more information or to file complaints about weight-loss products or programs

Food and Nutrition Information Center (FNIC)
National Agricultural Library
10301 Baltimore Blvd, Room 304
Beltsville, MD 20705-2351
301 504-5719

Answers questions concerning food and nutrition and provides database searches, bibliographies, and resource guides on a wide variety of food and nutrition topics.

National Arthritis and Musculoskeletal and Skin Diseases
Information Clearinghouse
Box AMS
9000 Rockville Pike
Bethesda, MD 20892
(301) 495-4484

National Cancer Institute
Office of Cancer Communications and Information Service
Building 31
Room 10A24
Bethesda, MD 20893
301) 496 5583
1 800 4-CANCER

For information on all cancers and diet, nutrition and the prevention of cancer

National Clearinghouse for Alcohol and Drug Abuse Information
(NCADI)
P. O. Box 2345
Rockville, MD 20847-2345
(800) 729-6686; (301) 468-2600

Central point within the Federal government for current print and audiovisual information about alcohol and other drugs. Publication for women include: Alcohol Alert #10; Alcohol and Women; Alcohol, Tobacco, and Other Drugs May Harm an Unborn; Women and Alcohol. A publications catalog is available.

National Dairy Council
    10255 West Higgins Road
    #900
    Rosemont, IL 60018-5616
    (708) 803-2000

    Provides nutrition education materials such as "Every Woman's Guide to Health and Nutrition", "Food and Activity Record", "Calcium: A Summary of Current Research-2nd edition". Request a Nutrition Education Materials Order Form. Minor charges. Some items available in spanish.

National Diabetes Information Clearinghouse (NDIC)
    1 Information Way
    Bethesda, MD 20892-3560
    (301) 654-3327

    Provides information to diabetic patients and provides materials on topics such as diabetes management and treatment, nutrition, dental care, insulin, and self-blood glucose monitoring.

National Heart, Lung, and Blood Institute (NHLBI)
    Information Center
    NHLBI Information Center
    P.O. Box 30105
    Bethesda, MD 20824-0105
    301) 251-1222

    Provides public and patient education materials on high blood pressure, cholesterol, smoking, obesity, and heart disease

National Institute on Aging (NIA) Information Center
    P.O. Box 8057
    Gaithersburg, MD 20898-8057
    (800) 222-2225

National Osteoporosis Foundation (NOF)
    1150 17th St. N.W.
    Suite 500
    Washington, D.C. 20036-4603
    202 223 2226

    For information on osteoporosis prevention and treatment. Several publications available.

National Mental Health Association (NMHA)
     Information Center
     1021 Prince Street
     Alexandria, VA 22314-2971
     (703) 684-7722
     (800) 969-6642

National Women's Health Network
     514 10th St N.W.
     #400
     Washington, DC 20004
     202) 347-1140

National Women's Health Resource Center (NWHRC)
     2440 M Street, N. W.
     Suite 325
     Washington, DC 20037
     (202) 293-6045

North American Menopause Society (NAMS)
     C/O University Hospitals of Cleveland
     Department of OB/GYN
     11100 Euclid Avenue
     Cleveland, OH 44106
     (216) 844-3334

     Provides information on a number of different topics which
     affect women during menopause and postmenopause.

Office of Disease Prevention and Health Promotion
     National Health Information Center (ONHIC)
     P.O. Box 1133
     Washington, DC 20013-1133
     (800) 336-4797; (301) 565-4167

     Helps the public and health professionals locate health
     information through identification of health information
     resources. A publications list is available.

Office of Research on Women's Health
    National Institutes of Health (NIH)
    9000 Rockville Pike
    Bldg 1 Room 201
    Bethesda, MD 20892-0161
    301 402 1770

    For background and information on studies and referrals to
    various NIH information offices

Office on Smoking and Health (OSH)
    Center for Chronic Disease Prevention and Health
    Promotion
    Centers for Disease Control and Prevention
    4770 Bufford Hwy N. E.
    Atlanta, GA 30341-3724
    (404) 488-5705

    Provides information on smoking cessation.

Older Women's League (OWL)
    666 11th Street, NW
    Suite 700
    Washington, DC 20001
    (202) 783-6686

Sex Information and Education Council of the U.S. (SIECUS)
    130 West 42nd Street
    Suite 350
    New York, NY 10036
    (212) 819-9770

Superintendent of Documents
    U.S. Government Printing Office
    Washington, DC 20402-9352
    (202) 512-1800

    Makes available many health-related publications from
    Government agencies. There are charges for publications.
    Write for a free copy of *U.S. Government Books and New
    Books* to receive information on what is available.

U. S. Department of Agriculture
Center for Nutrition Policy and Promotion
1120 20th St. N. W.
#200 North
Washington, DC 20036
(202) 418-2312

Reports results of research on food consumption, food composition, and dietary guidance in both technical and popular publications. A list of Department of Agriculture publications is available.

U.S. Department of Agriculture
Dietary Guidelines and Your Diet packet
(numbers HG-232-1 through HG-232-7)

Seven booklets which deal with avoiding too much fat, saturated fat, cholesterol, and too much sodium; also includes foods with adequate fiber and starch. Write to:
Superintendent of Documents, Government Printing Office, Washington, DC 20402; include payment of $4.50 and request stock number 001-000-04467-2.

U.S. Department of Health and Human Services
National Cancer Institute and National Heart Lung and Blood Institute.
Eating for Life (1988).
NIH Publication No. 88-3000.
Superintendent of Documents
U.S. Government Printing Office. Washington, DC 20402

Wider Opportunities for Women (WOW)
National Commission on Working Women
1325 G Street, NW
Washington, DC 20005
(202) 737-5764

References

INTRODUCTION

1. Utian, W. H., & Schiff, I. (1994). NAMS—Gallup survey on women's knowledge, information sources, and attitudes to menopause and hormone replacement therapy. *Menopause: The Journal of the American Menopause Society, 1,* 39–48.

CHAPTER ONE

1. U.S. Congress, Office of Technology Assessment. (May, 1992). *The menopause, hormone therapy, and women's health,* OTA-BP-BA-88, Washington, DC: U.S. Government Printing Office.

2. Deutsch, H. (1945). *The psychology of women, A psychoanalytical interpretation.* New York: Grune and Stratton.

3. Schlossberg, N. K. (1989). *Overwhelmed: Coping with life's ups and downs.* Lexington, MA: Lexington Books.

4. U.S. Department of Health and Human Services, Public Health Service, (Dec. 1992). *Menopause.* NIH Publication No. 92- 3466, Bethesda, MD: National Institutes of Health, National Institute on Aging.

5. McKinlay. S. M., & McKinlay, J. B. (1989). The impact of menopause and social factors on health. In C. B. Hammond, F. P. Hazeltine & I. Schiff (Eds.). *Menopause: Evaluation, treatment, and health concerns* (pp. 137–161). New York: Alan R. Liss.

6. Avis, N. E., & McKinlay, S. M. (1991). A longitudinal analysis of women's attitudes toward the menopause: Results from the Massachusetts Women's Health Study. *Maturitas, 13,* 65–79.

7. Speroff, L. (1994). The menopause: A signal for the future. In R. Lobo (Ed.). *Treatment of the postmenopausal woman: Basic and clinical aspects.* (pp 1–8). New York: Raven Press.

8. Plunkett, E. R., & Wolfe, B. M. (1992). Prolonged effects of a novel, low-dosage continuous progestin-cyclic estrogen replacement program in postmenopausal women. *Am J Obstet Gynecol, 166,* 1, 117–21.

CHAPTER TWO

1. U.S. Congress, Office of Technology Assessment. (May, 1992). *The menopause, hormone therapy, and women's health,* OTA-BP-BA-88, Washington, DC: U.S. Government Printing Office.

2. Utian, W. H. (1980). *Menopause in perspective: A guide to clinical practice.* New York: Appleton-Century-Croft.

3. Naftolin, F. (1994). The use of androgens. In R. Lobo (Ed.). *Treatment of the postmenopausal woman: Basic and clinical aspects.* (pp 91–94). New York: Raven Press.

4. Buckler, H. M., & Anderson, D. C. (1994). The perimenopausal state and incipient ovarian failure. In R. Lobo (Ed.). *Treatment of the postmenopausal woman: Basic and clinical aspects.* (pp 11–23). New York: Raven Press.

5. Herbst, A.L. et al. (1992). *Comprehensive gynecology* (2nd ed.). St. Louis: Mosby Year Book.

6. Kronenberg, F. (1994). Hot flashes. In R. Lobo (Ed.). *Treatment of the postmenopausal woman: Basic and clinical aspects.* (pp 97–117). New York: Raven Press.

7. Nachtigall, L. E., & Heilman-Rattner, J. (1991). *Estrogen,* (p.76). New York: Harper Perennial.

8. Palinkas, L. A., & Barrett-Connor, E. (1992). Estrogen use and depressive symptoms in postmenopausal women. *Obstetrics and Gynecology, 80*(1), 30–36.

9. Studd, J.W., & Smith, R. N. (1994). Estrogens and depression in women. *Menopause, 1,* 33–37.

References

10. U.S. Department of Health and Human Services, Public Health Service, (Dec. 1992). *Menopause.* NIH Publication No. 92–3466, Bethesda, MD: National Institutes of Health, National Institute on Aging.

11 Vliet, E. L., & Hutcheson-Davis, V. L. (1991). New perspectives on the relationship of hormone changes to affective disorders in the perimenopause. *NAACOG's Clinical Issues in Perinatal and Women's Health Nursing—Midlife Women's Health,* 2(4), 453–471.

12. Sherwin, B. B. (1994). Impact of the changing hormone milieu on psychological functioning. In R. Lobo (Ed.) *Treatment of the postmenopausal woman: Basic and clinical aspects.* (pp 119–127). New York: Raven Press.

13. Barrett-Connor, E., & Kritz-Silverstein, D. (1993). Estrogen replacement therapy and cognitive function in older women. *Journal of the American Medical Association, 269,* 2637–2641.

14. Limouzin-Lamothe, M. A., Mairon, N., Joyce, C. B., & LeGal, M. (1994.). Quality of life after the menopause: Influence of hormonal replacement therapy. *American Journal of Obstetrics and Gynecology, 170,* 618–624.

15. Regestein, Q. R. (1994). Menopausal aspects of sleep disturbance. In J. Lorrain, L. Plouffe Jr., V. Ravnikar, L. Speroff & N. Watts (Eds.). *Comprehensive management of menopause.* (pp 358–366). New York: Springer-Verlag.

16. Moore, D. E. (1992). Management of menopause. In M. A. Stenchever (Ed.) *Office gynecology* (pp 136–174). St. Louis: Mosby Year Book.

17. Sherwin, B. B. (1994). Sex hormones and psychological functioning in postmenopausal women. *Experimental Gerontology,* 29(3/4), 423–430.

18. Brincat, M., Moniz, C. F., Studd, J. W., et al (1983). Sex hormones and skin collagen content in postmenopausal women. *British Medical Journal, 287,* 1337.

19. Brincat, M., Moniz, C. F., Studd, J. W., Derby, A. J., Magos, A., Eumbery, G., & Versi, E. (1985). The long-term effects of the menopause and of administration of sex hormones

on skin collagen and skin thickness. *British Journal of Obstetrics and Gynaecology, 92,* 256–259.

20. Brincat, M., Versi, E. Moniz, C. F., Magos, A., DeTrafford, J., & Studd, J. W. (1987). Skin collagen changes in postmenopausal women receiving different regimens of oestrogen therapy. *Obstetrics and Gynecology, 70*(6), 840–845.

21. Formosa, M., Brincat, M. P., Cardozo, L. D., & Studd, J. W. (1994). Collagen: The significance in skin, bones, and bladder. In R. Lobo (Ed.) *Treatment of the postmenopausal woman: Basic and clinical aspects.* (pp 143–151). New York: Raven Press.

22. National Institutes of Health, National Heart, Lung and Blood Institute. (1994). The cardiovascular health of women. *Heart Memo.* Bethesda, MD: National Heart, Lung and Blood Institute Information Center.

23. Gotto, A. M., Jr., & Hoffman, A. S. (1993). Lipid metabolism and menopause. In J. Lorrain, L. Plouffe Jr., V. Ravnikar, J. Speroff, & N. Watts (Eds.), *Comprehensive management of menopause* (pp. 215–226). New York: Springer-Verlag.

24. Heymsfield, S. B., Gallagher, D., Poehlman, E. T., Wolper, C., Nonas, K., Nelson, D., & Wang, Z. (1994). Menopausal changes in body composition and energy expenditure. *Experimental Gerontology, 29*(3/4), 377–389.

25. Aloia, J. F., McGowan, D. B., Vaswani, A. N., Ross, P., & Cohn, S. H. (1991). Relationship of menopause to skeletal and muscle mass. *American Journal of Clinical Nutrition, 53,* 1378–1383.

26. Forbes, G. B. (Ed.). (1987). *Human body composition: Growth, aging, nutrition, and activities.* New York: Springer-Verlag.

CHAPTER THREE

1. National Osteoporosis Foundation. (1994). *Osteoporosis facts: Financial costs.* Washington, DC: Author.

2. National Osteoporosis Foundation. (1994). *Fast facts on osteoporosis.* Washington, DC: Author.

References

3. Peck, W. A. (1990). Estrogen therapy after menopause. *Journal of the American Medical Women's Association, 45*(3), 87–90.

4. Barrett-Connor, E., Chang, J. C., & Edelstein, S. L. (1994). Coffee-associated osteoporosis offset by daily milk consumption. *Journal of the American Medical Association, 271,* 280– 283.

5. Holbrook, T. L., & Connor-Barrett, E. (1993). A prospective study of alcohol consumption and bone mineral density. *British Medical Journal, 306,* 1506–1509.

6. Chestnut, C. H. (1992). Methods and role of bone densitometry in the estrogen-deficient woman. In D. P. Swartz (Ed.). *Hormone replacement therapy* (pp. 65–78). Baltimore: Williams & Wilkins.

7. Marcus, R., Christiansen, C., Johnston, C. C., & Lindsay, R. B. (1991). *Osteoporosis update: Highlights from an international conference.* Philadelphia: Wyeth-Ayerst Laboratories.

8. National Osteoporosis Foundation. (1995). *Current perspectives on diagnosis, prevention, and treatment of osteoporosis.* Washington, DC: Author

9. Avioli, L. V. (1995). New nasal spray Calcitonin for the treatment of postmenopausal osteoporosis. *Osteoporosis Report, 2*(3), 4–5.

10. National Osteoporosis Foundation. (1994). *Drugs in the prevention and treatment of osteoporosis.* Washington, DC: Author.

11. National Osteoporosis Foundation. (1994). *Calcium: Important at every age.* Washington, DC: Author.

12. Dairy Council Digest. (1995). *Calcium sources: The case for foods first, 66*(1), Rosemont, IL: National Dairy Council.

13. U. S. Department of Agriculture & U. S. Department of Health and Human Services. (1990). *Dietary guidelines for Americans.* (3rd ed.). Home and Garden Bulletin No. 232. Hyattsville, MD: Author.

14. National Osteoporosis Foundation. (1995). *Current per-*

spectives on diagnosis, prevention, and treatment of osteoporosis. Washington, DC: Author

15. National Osteoporosis Foundation. (1994). *Exercise for your bone health.* Washington, DC: Author.

16. Ettinger, B., & Drinkwater, B. L. (1992). Calcium and exercise: Alternatives or adjuncts to estrogen in preventing osteoporosis. In D. P. Swartz (Ed.). *Hormone replacement therapy* (pp.79–108), Baltimore, MD.: Williams and Wilkins.

17. Jacobson, P. C., Beaver, W., Grubb, S. A., Taft, T. N., & Talmage, R. V. (1984). Bone density in women: College athletes and older athletic women, *Journal of Orthopedic Research, 2,* 328–332.

18. McBean, L. D. (1992). Calcium and osteoporosis: New insights. *Dairy Council Digest, 63*(1), Rosemont, IL: National Dairy Council.

19. U.S. Congress, Office of Technology Assessment. (May, 1992). *The menopause, hormone therapy, and women's health,* OTA-BP-BA-88, Washington, DC: U.S. Government Printing Office.

20. Update: Estrogen (1995, April). *Lunar News,* 18–19. Madison, WI: Lunar Corporation.

21. National Osteoporosis Foundation. (1994). *Bone health tips for women in midlife.* Washington, DC: Author.

22. National Osteoporosis Foundation. (1994). *Bone health tips for older men and women.* Washington, DC: Author.

23. National Osteoporosis Foundation. (1995). *Bone basics for teens.* Washington, DC: Author.

24. National Osteoporosis Foundation. (1994). *Bone health tips for teens.* Washington, DC: Author.

25. National Osteoporosis Foundation. (1994). *Bone health tips for men of all ages.* Washington, DC: Author.

26. Shangold, M. M. (1994). Menstruation and Menstrual disorders. In M. M. Shangold & G. Mirkin (Eds.), *Women and exercise* (pp. 152–171). Philadelphia: F. A. Davis Company.

27. Dent, C. E. (1973).Keynote Address: Problems in meta-

bolic bone disease, In B. Frame, A. M. Parfitt, & H. E. Duncan, (Eds) *Clinical aspects of metabolic bone disease. Amsterdam: Excerpta Medica.*

28. Klibanski, A. (1994). Bone loss in young women with anorexia nervosa. *Osteoporosis Report, 10*(2), 2–3.

CHAPTER FOUR

1. American Heart Association. (1995). *Heart and stroke facts: 1995 statistical supplement.* Author.

2. LaRosa, J. C. (1995). Has HRT come of age? *The Lancet, 345,* 76–77.

3. National Heart, Lung and Blood Institute. (1994). *Heart disease and women: Are you at risk?* (NIH Publication No. 94-3654). Bethesda, MD: National Institutes of Health.

4. Sandmaier, M. (1992). *The healthy heart handbook.* National Heart, Lung and Blood Institute. (NIH Publication No. 92-2720). Washington, DC: Superintendent of Documents.

5. Jacobs, D. R. Jr., Melbane, I. L., & Bangdiwala, S. I. (1990). High density lipoprotein cholesterol as a predictor of car-diovascular disease mortality in men and women: The follow-up study of the Lipid Research Clinics Prevalence Study. *American Journal of Epidemiology, 131,* 32.

6. Larosa, J. C. (1994). Management of postmenopausal women who have hyperlipidemia. *The American Journal of Medicine, 96,* (suppl 6A), 19S–23S.

7. Levin, E. G., Miller, V. T., Muesing, R. A., Stoy, D. G., Balm, T. K., & LaRosa, J. C. (1990). Comparison of psyllium hydrophilic mucilloid and cellulose as adjuncts to a prudent diet in the treatment of mild to moderate hypercholesterolemia. *Archives of Internal Medicine, 150,* 1822 –1827.

8. Hunninghake, D. B., Miller, V. T., LaRosa, J. C., Kinosian, B., Brown, V., Howard, W. J., DiSerio, F. J., & O'Connor, R. R. (1994). Hypocholesterolemic effects of a dietary fiber supplement. *American Journal of Clinical Nutrition, 59,* 1050–1054.

9. National Heart, Lung and Blood Institute. (1994). *Heart disease and women: Getting physical* , (NIH Publication No. 94-3656). Bethesda, MD: National Institutes of Health.

10. LaRosa, J. C. (1994). Management of postmenopausal women who have hyperlipidemia. *The American Journal of Medicine, 96,* (suppl 6A), 19S–23S.

11. LaRosa, J. C. (1995). Has HRT come of age? *Lancet, 345* (8942), 76–77.

12. Taylor, P. A., & Ward, A. (1993). Women, high-density lipoprotein cholesterol, and exercise. *Archives of Internal Medicine, 153,* 1178–1184.

13. Manson, J. E., Stampfer, M. J., Colditz, G. A., Willett, W. C., Rosner, B., Speizer, F. E., & Hennekens, C. H. (1991). A prospective study of aspirin use and primary prevention of cardiovascular disease in women. *Journal of the American Medical Association. 266*(4), 521–527.

CHAPTER FIVE

1. Harlap, S. (1992). The benefits and risks of hormone replacement therapy: An epidemiologic overview. *American Journal of Obstetrics and Gynecology, 166*(6), (suppl. part 2), 1986–1992.

2. Ellerington, M. C., Whitcroft, S. J., & Whitehead, M. I. (1994). Therapeutic and preventive aspects of estrogen and progesterone therapy. In J. Lorrain, L. Plouffe Jr., V. Ravnikar, L. Speroff & N. Watts (Eds.). *Comprehensive management of menopause.* (pp 269–285). New York: Springer-Verlag.

3. Naftolin, F. (1994). The use of androgens. In R. Lobo (Ed.). *Treatment of the postmenopausal woman: Basic and clinical aspects.* (pp 91–94). New York: Raven Press.

4. Plouffe, L. Jr., & Cohen, D. P. (1994). The role of androgens in menopausal hormone replacement therapy. In J. Lorrain, L. Plouffe Jr., V. Ravnikar, L. Speroff & N. Watts (Eds.). *Comprehensive management of menopause.* (pp 297–308). New York: Springer-Verlag.

5. Stumpf, P. (1992). Estrogen replacement therapy: Current

regimens. In D. P. Swartz (Ed.). *Hormone replacement therapy* (pp.171–190), Baltimore, MD.: Williams and Wilkins.

6. Samsioe, G. N., & Mattsson, L. (1994). Regimens for today and the future. In R. Lobo (Ed.). *Treatment of the postmenopausal woman: Basic and clinical aspects.* (pp 421–426). New York: Raven Press.

7. PEPI Trial Group. (1995). Effects of estrogen or estrogen/progestin regimens on heart disease risk factors in postmenopausal women. *Journal of the American Medical Association, 273,* 199–208.

8. Healy, B. (1995). PEPI in perspective: Good answers spawn pressing questions. (editorial) *Journal of the American Medical Association, 273,* 240–241

9. News Briefs (1995, March/April). Initial results of the PEPI trial. *Menopause Management, 24.*

10. Shoupe, D., & Mishell, D. R. (1994). Contraindications to hormone replacement. In R. Lobo (Ed.). *Treatment of the postmenopausal woman: Basic and clinical aspects.* (pp 415–418). New York: Raven Press.

11. Watts, N. B. (1994). Complicated and controversial considerations regarding estrogen replacement therapy. In J. Lorrain, L. Plouffe Jr., V. Ravnikar, L. Speroff & N. Watts (Eds.). *Comprehensive management of menopause.* (pp 395–397).   New York: Springer-Verlag.

12. Chu, J., Schweid, A. I., & Weiss, N. S. (1982). Survival among women with endometrial cancer: A comparison of estrogen users and nonusers. *N. Engl J Med, 143,* 569–73.

13. American Cancer Society. (1995). *Cancer facts and figures.* 10, Author.

14. Hulka, B. S., Liu, D. T. & Lininger, R. A. (1994). Steroid hormones and risk of breast cancer. *Cancer Supplement,* 74(3), 1111–1124.

15. Dupont, W. D., Page, D. L., Rogers, L. W., & Parl, F. F. (1989). Influence of exogenous estrogens, proliferative breast disease, and other variables on breast cancer risk. *A Cancer Journal for Clinicians, 63,* 948.

16. Colditz, G. A., Hankinson, S. E., Hunter, D. J., Willett, W. C., Manson, J. E., Stampfer, M. J., Hennekens, C., Rosner, B., & Speizer, F. E. (1995). The use of estrogens and progestins and the risk of breast cancer in postmenopausal women. *The New England Journal of Medicine, 332*(24), 1590–1593.

17. Eden, J. A., Bush, T., Nand, S., & Wren, B. G. (1995). A case-control study of combined continuous estrogen-progestin replacement therapy among women with a personal history of breast cancer. Menopause: *The Journal of the North American Menopause Society, 2,* 67–72.

18. U.S. Department of Health and Human Services. (1994). *Quality mammography/A woman's guide: Things to know about quality mammograms.* (AHCPR Publication No. 95-0634). Rockville, MD: Author

19. Landau, C., Cyr, M. G., & Moulton, A. W. (1994). *The complete book of menopause.* (p.54). New York: Grosset/Putnam Book.

20. Teaf, N. L., & Wiley, K. W. (1995). *Perimenopause: Preparing for the change.* (pp. 134, 135). Rocklin, CA: Prima.

21. Setchell, K. D. R. (1994, September). *Dietary estrogens: Metabolism and physiological effects in humans.* Paper presented at the meeting of the North American Menopause Society, Washington, DC.

22. Aldercreutz, H. (1994, September). *Lignans and isoflavonoids:Epidemiology and prevention of cancer and other diseases.* Paper presented at the meeting of the North American Menopause Society, Washington, DC.

23. Mirkin, G. (1991). Estrogen in yams. *Journal of American Medical Association, 265,* 912.

24. Barnard, N. D. (1994). Natural progesterone. *Prevention & Nutrition,* Spring, 11–13.

25. Kronenberg, F. (1995). Alternative therapies: New opportunities for menopause research. *Menopause, 2*(1), 1–2.

26. Freeman, S. (1995). Menopause without HRT: Complimentary therapies. *Contemporary Nurse Practitioner, 1*(1), 40–49.

27. Andrews, W. C. (1995). The transitional years and beyond. *Obstetrics & Gynecology, 85,* 1–5.

28. Contraception: When is it safe to stop. *VIA.* (Dec. 1994).15–16.

CHAPTER SIX

1. U. S. Department of Agriculture & U. S. Department of Health and Human Services. (1990). *Dietary guidelines for Americans.* (3rd ed.). Home and Garden Bulletin No. 232. Hyattsville, MD: Author.

2. U. S. Department of Agriculture. (1992). *The food guide pyramid.* Home and Garden Bulletin No. 252. Hyattsville, MD: Author.

3. Wilfley, D. E., Grilo, C. M., & Brownell, K. D. (1994). Exercise and regulation of body weight. In M. M. Shangold & G. Mirkin (Eds.), *Women and exercise* (pp. 27–54). Philadelphia: F. A. Davis Company.

4. Department of Health and Human Services. (1992). *The facts about weight loss products and programs.* DHHS Publication NO. (FDA) 92-1189.

5. Papazian, R. (1991). *An FDA guide to dieting.* DHHS (FDA)92- 1188. Rockville, MD: Food and Drug Administration.

6. Diplock, A. T. (1991). Antioxidant nutrients and disease prevention: An overview. *American Journal of Clinical Nutrition, 53,* 189–192S.

7. Hennekens, C. H. (Ed.). (1994). Health promotion and disease prevention: The role of antioxidant vitamins. *American Journal of Medicine, 97*(3A), 1S–28S.

8. Hankinson, S. E., & Stampfer, M. J. (1994). All that glitters is not beta carotene. *Journal of the American Medical Association, 272,* 1455–1456.

9. Seddon, J. M., Ajani, U. A., Sperduto, R. D., Hiller, R., Blair, N., Burton, T. C., Farber, M. D., Gragoudas, E. S., Haller, J., Miller, D. T., Yannuzzi, L. A., & Willett, W. (1994). Dietary carotenoids, vitamins A, C, and E, and advanced age-related mac-

ular degeneration. *Journal of the American Medical Association, 272,* 1413–1420.

10. Morris, D. L., Kritchevsky, S. B., & Davis, C. E. (1994). Serum carotenoids and coronary heart disease. *Journal of the American Medical Association, 272,* 1439–1441.

11. Zusy, M. J., & Lakatta, P. (1992). Nurses: Determining the future of women's health, *The Nursing Spectrum,* 2(21), 10–11.

12. Buring, J. E. (1992). Personal communication. Women's Health Study. Brigham and Women's Hospital and Harvard Medical School. Boston, MA.

13. U.S. Department of Health and Human Services. National Institutes of Health, National Heart, Lung and Blood Institute. American Heart Association (1993). *Exercise and your heart: A guide to physical activity.* NIH Publication No. 93-1677. U.S. Government Printing Office.

14. Maryland Department of Health and Mental Hygiene. (1983). *Getting fit your way: A self-paced fitness guide.* Baltimore, MD: Author.

15. The President's Council on Physical Fitness and Sports. (1992). Walking for Exercise and Pleasure. GPO: 1992 0-326-101. Washington, DC: Superintendent of Documents, U.S. Government Printing Office.

16. Bachmann, G. A., & Grill, J. (1987). Exercise in the postmenopausal woman. *Geriatric, 42,* 75–85.

17. Active lifestyle may be all that's necessary. (1995). *Advance,* 28A.

18. Dairy Council of Greater Metropolitan Washington, Inc. (1995). *Working on Wellness,* 6(1), Reston, VA: Author.

19. National Osteoporosis Foundation (Summer, 1995). The use of exercise machines. *Osteoporosis Report, 11*(2). Washington, DC: Author

20. LaPerriere, A., Ironson, G., Antoni, M. H., Schneiderman, N., Klimas, N., & Fletcher, M. A. (1994). Exercise and psychoneuroimmunology. *Medicine and Science in Sports and Exercise. 26,* 182–190.

21. Mackinnon, L. T. (1994). Current challenges and future expectations in exercise immunology: Back to the future. *Medicine and Science in Sports Medicine, 26,* 191–194.

22. Nieman, D. C. (1994). Exercise, upper respiratory tract infection, and the immune system. *Medicine and Science in Sports and Exercise, 26,* 128–139.

23. Girdano-Dusek, D. (1979). Stress reduction through physical activity. In D. A. Girdano & G. S. Everly (Eds.), *Controlling stress and tension: A holistic approach* (pp.220–231). Englewood Cliffs, NJ: Prentice-Hall.

CHAPTER SEVEN

1. U.S. Congress, Office of Technology Assessment. (May, 1992). *The menopause, hormone therapy, and women's health,* OTA-BP-BA-88, Washington, DC: U.S. Government Printing Office.

2. NIH. (1992). *Report of the National Institutes of Health: Opportunities for research on women's health* (summary report), Office of Research on Women's Health, U.S. Dept. of Health and Human Services, National Institutes of Health (NIH), NIH publication NO. 92-3457, September 1992. S/N 017-040-00522-9. Pittsburgh: Superintendent of Documents, P. O. Box 371954

3. Paganini-Hill, A. (1994). Morbidity and mortality changes with estrogen replacement therapy. In R. Lobo Ed.). *Treatment of the postmenopausal woman: Basic and clinical aspects.* (pp 300–404). New York: Raven Press.

4. Henderson, B. D., Paganini-Hill, A., & Ross, R.K. (1991). Decreased mortality in users of estrogen replacement therapy. *Arch Intern Med, 151,* 75–78.

5. Colditz, G. A., Hankinson, S. E., Hunter, D. J., Willett, W. C., Manson, J. E., Stampfer, M. J., Hennekens, C., Rosner, B., & Speizer, F. E. (1995). The use of estrogens and progestins and the risk of breast cancer in postmenopausal women. *The New England Journal of Medicine, 332*(24), 1590–1593.

6. Bush, T. (1995, September). Breast cancer and long-term hormone replacement therapy. *Long-term HRT balancing the risk:*

Benefit equation. North American Menopause Society Colloquium special pre-conference program, San Francisco, California.

7. PEPI Trial Group. (1995). Effects of estrogen or estrogen/progestin regimens on heart disease risk factors in post-menopausal women. *Journal of the American Medical Association, 273,* 199–208.

8. Healy, B. (1995). PEPI in perspective: Good answers spawn pressing questions. (editorial) *Journal of the American Medical Association, 273,* 240–241

9. Greendale, G. A., & Bush, T. (1995, September). *Hormonal effects on bone mineral density in the spine and hip: Results from the postmenopausal estrogen/progestin intervention trial.* North American Menopause Society Annual Meeting, San Francisco, California.

10. Zusy, M. J., & Lakatta, P. (1992). Nurses: Determining the future of women's health, *The Nursing Spectrum, 2*(21), 10–11.

11. Buring, J. E. (1992). Personal communication. Women's Health Study. Brigham and Women's Hospital and Harvard Medical School. Boston, MA.

12. Food and Drug Administration Medical Bulletin (Dec. 1993). Women in Clinical Trials. Vol. 23, No. 3 (pp 2–4), Department of Health & Human Services. Public Health Service, Food and Drug Administration (HFI-42), Rockville MD.

Index

NOTES

NOTES

NOTES

NOTES

NOTES

NOTES

NOTES

NOTES

NOTES

NOTES

NOTES

NOTES

NOTES

NOTES

NOTES

NOTES

HEALTH LEADERSHIP ASSOCIATES, INC
Book Order Form
for additional books for a friend or colleague

Please print or type

Name _____

Address _____

Street _____

City _____ State _____ Zip _____

Tel. Home _____ Work _____

	Quantity	Price	Total
Today and Tomorrow's Woman			
Menopause: Before and After	_____	@ $19.95	_____
		Subtotal	_____

Maryland residents add 5% sales tax _____

Shipping $5.00 for one book _____

$1.00 for each additional book _____

Total _____

Mail this order form, with your credit card or P.O. number or check (US Funds) to: Health Leadership Associates, Inc.
P.O. Box 59153
Potomac, MD 20859

Call toll-free **1-800-435-4775** with your VISA, Mastercard or purchase order number

Fax this order form or your purchase order to **301-983-2693**

For purchase orders, P.O. # _____
(attach copy of purchase order)

Please charge my   ☐ Visa   ☐ MC

Credit Card # _____

Expiration Date _____

Print Name _____

Signature _____

For orders of 10 or greater call 1-800-435-4775
(All prices subject to change without notice)